PA[T...]
TO HEALING

A GUIDE TO HERBS, AYURVEDA, DREAMBODY, & SHAMANISM

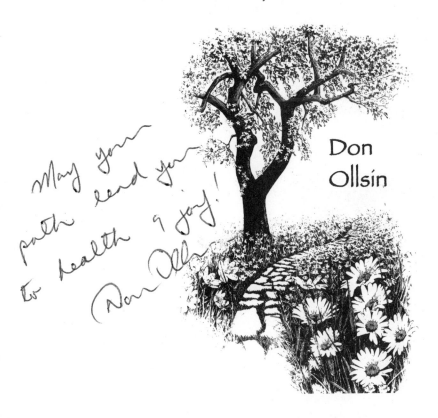

Don
Ollsin

May your path lead you to health & joy!

Don Ollsin

Aquiline Communications
Victoria, BC, Canada

All the information in *Pathways to Healing* is based on the experiences and research of the author and other professional healers. This information is shared with the understanding that you accept complete responsibility for your own health and well-being. You have a unique body and mind. The action of every remedy is also unique. Health care is full of variables. The result of any treatment suggested herein cannot always be anticipated and never guaranteed. The author and publisher are not responsible for any adverse effects or consequences resulting from the use of any remedies, procedures, or preparations included in *Pathways to Healing*. Consult your inner guidance, knowledgeable friends, and trained healers in addition to this book.

Published by Aquiline Communications
Aquiline Communications books are distributed by
North Atlantic Books, P.O. Box 12327, Berkeley, CA 94712

Previously published by Aquiline Communications as *Herbal Healing Journey* (ISBN 1-894287-01-0)

Cover design by Paula Morrison
Illustrations by Soren Henrich

Printed in the United States of America

Library of Congress Cataloging-in-Publication Data
Ollsin, Don, 1946–
  Pathways to healing : a guide to herbs, ayurveda, dreambody, and shamanism / by Don Ollsin
    p. cm.
  Includes index.
  ISBN 1-58394-011-1 (pbk. : alk. paper)
  1. Alternative medicine. 2. Herbs—Therapeutic use. I Title.
R733.O44 1999
615.5—dc21   99-051552

1 2 3 4 5 6 7 8 9 / 05 04 03 02 01 00

Table of Contents

"Tell me and I will forget.

Teach me and I will remember.

Involve me and I will learn."

Benjamin Franklin

ACKNOWLEDGEMENTS

I would like to thank Sandy for her love, support, continual encouragement and fine editing. Our three children, Melissa, Jonn and Brooke for keeping me connected to the magic (dreamworld) and the mundane (ordinary world). My mother who showed me a functional model of how to live in this world. And my father whose dysfunction, prompted my search for wholeness.

My friends: Ken Bloomfield for his wise counsel and editorial comments. Stan Tomandl for his support, processing skills and positive feedback. Chris Carless for his long hours, creative wit and continual support and encouragement. Carmen Lane for her excellent typesetting and Paula Morrison for the cover design and Soren Henrich for his creative illustrations.

My teachers: Ellen White for her friendship, guidance and shamanic teachings. Kirpal Singh for his continual support, guidance and direction in the spiritual world. Dr. John Christopher for his trail blazing. Norma Myers for her wild - woman ways. Rosemary Gladstar for her warmth and support. Susun Weed for her guidance, encouragement and speaking her truth. Ryan Drum for his friendship and wildcrafting teachings. Robbie Svoboda for opening the doors of Ayurveda for me. Dorothy Maclean who talked to devas and passed on her inspiration and encourgement to me. Arnie Mindell who taught me how to experience, follow and grow through the dreaming body.

Every student and client I have had the privilege of being with. All of the graduates of the Herbal Healing Journey.

The Earth, Water, Wind and Fire and all their gifts as well as the Plant Beings and especially the Oak Deva.

Don Ollsin

FOREWORD

I have a treasured memory of Don Ollsin and I at the onset of our friendship moving warily towards each other over many months. Feeling each other out, a powerful affirmation of exercise 61 in this book. What became clear as we became more comfortable with each other was that, as herbalists and teachers, we were breaking away from rigid traditions in our work. I am passionately concerned with education, the process of learning, and the values that are conveyed just as much as the information. So is Don. He brings a remarkable understanding of learning as a life process and a skill in setting the scene whereby people can gain understanding, insight and self-awareness as well as information. He showed me the value of asking students questions and creating an environment where they can find their answers. I see Don as a teacher, coach and guide as well as an informer.

Since those early days we have become collaborators and I have had the immense pleasure and privilege to be invited to co-facilitate with Don in some of the courses he teaches. His knowledge is vast yet rooted in his search for deeper questions that will reveal new answers. This process has always led us to new ground, always searching, listening to our inner wisdom and guidance, connecting our knowledge of healing and learning. From it we have both been richer.

For Don his work with herbs, nature and his own inner world is a personal journey, the fruits of which he shares with clients and students and has for over twenty-five years.

The great teachings call us to "know ourselves, love our neighbour and do good works" with one startling omission that Don provides in the Herbal Healing Journey. He shows us how.

Rowan Hamilton. Herbalist. MNIMH MSCS Dip Phyt.

PREFACE

Welcome to the Pathways to Healing. This book is a journey of the self to the Self. It is a circular or spiral path circumambulating the Self. I am Don Ollsin and I was born in Assinaboia, Saskatchewan in 1946. My family moved to Vancouver, B.C. in 1954. In 1969, I travelled to India, where I lived, studied and meditated for six months. Afterward I returned to the West Coast and started various businesses - i.e. Health Food Restaurant, Natural Food Store and eventually, a Herbal Dispensary called Self Heal Herbs in Victoria, in 1976. I sold it in 1994 and am currently teaching, consulting and writing.

I work with herbs, plant devas, dreams, processes, elemental forces and natural medicines with clients and students. I have been sharing and building my repertoire of knowledge since 1969. I practice herbology, medicine-making, iridology, reflexology, shamanism and counselling. I use process-oriented psychology tools in my work. I am an active student of the dream world.

Don's Dream. *In this dream I come into a town and I ask where Carl Jung (one of the foremost founders of depth psychology) lives. I am directed to an apartment complex. I arrive at his door and with apprehension, I knock. His wife answers the door and leads me into the kitchen and departs. I stand there alone until Carl comes into the room. He looks at me and asks, "What are you doing with your life?" I begin to tell him that I am studying Dreambody with Arnold Mindell but he interrupts me. "I said, what are you doing? What do you have to offer to the world?"*

I remember two strong vivid awakenings that occurred around ages nine and thirteen. The first was in primary school. A teacher mentioned that the ancients had an archaic belief in the four elements. I remember experiencing a cloud of knowing enveloping me. I awoke in it and looked around wondering where I was and what was I being taught? In my previous world of knowledge, the four elements were fundamental to a precise and dynamic understanding of the world. Some deep part of me challenged the information being fed to me. As I looked around the classroom everything looked foreign to me, the walls, the windows and the desks. I remained in that heightened state for another fifteen minutes. It lingers in the present and guides me in this present work. I was approximately nine years old at the time.

My second awakening occurred when I was thirteen. I was sitting in my sister's car waiting for her. I was lost in deep thought as she approached the old Chevrolet. I didn't hear her open the door. She looked at me and inquired, "What are you doing? *Meditating?*" The word *meditating* invoked the most pleasant feeling that touched my spirit and spread throughout my body like internal goose bumps. I looked at her in dazed wonderment. "What does *meditation* mean?" I asked. In that moment

I knew that I knew better than her what meditation meant. By the age of nineteen I was actively pursuing the process of meditation. By twenty-two I was meditating three to six hours a day in an ashram in India under the guidance of Kirpal Singh, a true Master of the art and science of meditation. Through his grace and guidance I experience the incredible depths and joys that meditation brings. It has helped me immensely in my understanding of nature and her marvellous secrets.

I have studied personally with many teachers. Some of them include Kirpal Singh (Indian Mystic), Ellen White (Coast Salish Shaman), Stan Tomandl (Process Oriented Psychologist), Bernard Jensen (Nutritionist), Dr. Robbie Svoboda (Ayurvedic Doctor and Teacher), Dr. John Christopher (Herbalist), Eunice Ingham (Founder of Reflexology), Rolling Thunder (Medicine man), Dorothy Maclean (One of the founding members of Findhorn), Arnold Mindell (Founder of Process Oriented Psychology), and many others too numerous to mention.

I have conducted the intensive course, the Herbal Healing Journey, more than 17 times now. It includes experiential learning about herbs, healing, ayurveda, working with body symptoms using process-oriented psychology and shamanism. It has now evolved into a nine month course embracing home study and weekend practicums (see back of book).

I developed the exercises and accumulated the knowledge for this book over the last thirty years. The book is designed so that much of the learning comes from within yourself using the "do this" exercises to guide and support you.

My shamanic teacher, Ellen White, encourages us to think as **we**. We include: myself, my partner and editor Sandy, my children, my ancestors, my adopted grandmother Ellen White, my adopted grandfather Kirpal Singh, my friend Chris Carless, my buddy Stan Tomandl, my teachers, my students, my friends, my co-workers, the plant people, the elements, the ocean, the devas, the many beings from the spirit world. In Ellen's world we are connected to all life. Nothing lives in isolation.

Carl Jung introduced me to the idea that our symptoms and illnesses are very important circumstances deeply connected to our growth, not meaningless pathological symptoms. When we take the time and effort to listen, decipher and act on our symptoms they can be rich in meaning, full of information and offer new directions, attitudes or solutions.

You may want to ask yourself, " **What is right about this situation or symptom?**" By changing our questioning from what is wrong to what is right we may activate a new set of answers or solutions.

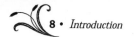

Healing Journey Goals

☐ My goal in writing this book is to offer you **tools and knowledge to increase your awareness that may initiate transformation in yourself and your life.**
I have designed the exercises for optimum learning based on the latest research in education.

☐ I want to share with you in an experiential way the **wonders and magic** of herbs, nature and life. If your life is changed in any small way for the better then my goal will be achieved and my heart will be happier.

☐ My goal of connecting your learning and wellness practices to the flow of the seasons is to connect you to a natural flow that is consistent, stable and defined.

Do This!

Exercise 1 • *Healing Journey Goals*

Answer the following questions.

• What do you want to get out of this book?

• Is there anything that you want to heal or change?

• Do you want to help others? How would you imagine doing that?

• Is there anything that would keep you from completing this course? What do you imagine it might be? What changes might you make to prevent this from happening?

• Preferably, discuss your goals and potential obstacles with a friend. Did anything new come out of the discussion?

"No favorable wind blows for a ship that has no port."

Personal Healing Myth

PERSONAL MYTH:

A strong experience that may create a pattern that tends to repeat itself.

PERSONAL EXAMPLE:

I remember being very sick when I was in grade five. I vomited out the contents of my stomach, then retched up bile and then had the dry heaves. It feels now like I was mostly alone. I did not go to the doctor. The only medicine I remember taking was some ginger ale.

I am sharing this with you to illustrate how it possibly shaped my **personal myth around healing**. Let's analyze it for fun and learning. Firstly, I was alone, so I obviously started developing the philosophy of **self-healing**. Secondly, the illness followed its own course, therefore since I got better I learned to **trust in the healing power of my body**.

The only medicine I used was Ginger Ale which is an **herbal beverage**. Ginger is an herb that I still like to use, although now I take Ginger tincture or strong Ginger tea. Ginger links many of us to our childhoods. That powerful childhood experience probably influenced my **interest in herbs**. More healing experience memories may present themselves at another time, but for now I will work with the one my memory offered.

"The child is father to the man" William Wordsworth

Do This!

Exercise 2 • *Healing Myth*

Recall your earliest memory of being ill.

- What was the illness like?

- What was going on in your life at the time?

- Who was with you?

- Where were you?

- How were you treated?

- How did you get better?

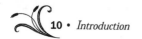

This may have set up a pattern for getting sick and how you deal with sickness. Think about other times that you have been sick. See if they have any similarities to the one you just recorded.

Pay attention to all of the different factors involved the next time you get sick. If you notice a pattern you may want to do something different with it, or at the very least follow the process with more awareness.

CHILDHOOD DREAM:

A strong recurring dream or strong memory that affected us during our childhood. Some may have been disturbing while others may have been exhilarating.

Do This!

Exercise 3 • *Childhood Dream*

Reflect back to your early childhood to find the first strong dream that you remember. Mine is "I am sitting in a very large building. It is dim in the building. I sit on the ground. A huge rope hangs down and swings hypnotically, back and forth." The strong part of the dream is the feeling that it evokes. I loved and feared that dream as it repeated itself often during my childhood.

When you have found your dream or memory spend time meditating on it. Maybe draw it, preferably in colour (big crayons are great) and write down any important words that capture the energy of the dream. Meditate on it again and pay attention to any feelings it evokes. Expand those feelings into small movements. Slowly increase the movements by increasing their range and tempo to the extent that is comfortable. Movement is challenging but often rewarding. If you have a willing partner then discuss the dream with them.

• Draw your childhood dream.

Contacting Your Inner Healer

This is an excellent exercise that I adapted from the book "Writing from the Body" by John Lee. His exercise is called meeting the inner artist. You can use this format for contacting different parts of yourself. Find out how they are doing and begin building a relationship with them. For the purpose of this work we will focus on the inner healer.

Do This!

Exercise 4 • *Inner Healer*

Find a place where you will be comfortable to spend some inner time. Relax and let your attention gently turn inward. Allow your attention to move toward the place where your healer lives. Search for the door that leads to where s/he lives. Observe what the door looks like. Ask if you can come in? When the healer appears, ask how they are doing? Do they need anything? Do they have anything to share with you? How could you foster the relationship? When you are finished, say goodbye and take a few minutes to reflect on the experience before drawing and writing about it.

- What is the door made of?

- Is it open or closed?

- Is the door used frequently or hardly at all?

- What does your inner healer look like?

- Did they need anything or have anything to share with you?

- Draw the experience: drawing sometimes helps to access other parts of ourselves.

- Record your experience.

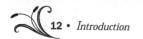

Healing Journey Guidelines

*"Enjoyable activities have **clear goals**, **stable rules** and **inspired challenges** well matched to **skills**." — from the book, "Flow"*

☐ Move toward **solutions**. Put most of your attention on the solution.

☐ Do all the **exercises** at least once. There is no right or wrong way to do the exercises, only personal experience and creative growth. Whatever you experience is valid. You may benefit from the repetition of some exercises until you become familiar with the technique. The exercises engage skills you may use to develop new ways of living and working.

☐ You may want to enlist the **support** of a friend or partner to share your experiences. Support is one of the 4 pillars (knowledgable healer, right medicine, patient cooperation) of healing. I learned through periods of isolation and suffering that I need support. Now I actively seek support and I am continually learning how to support others.

☐ We perceive life through our senses. By increasing our sensory perceptions we enlarge our experience of living and enrich our sense of aliveness. Whenever you feel spaced out or lost, **use your senses** to bring you back. Smell what you are smelling. See what you are seeing. Hear what you are hearing. Feel the sensation that you are feeling.

☐ Only consume as much as you can **digest**, physically, mentally, emotionally and spiritually. Some material may be totally new to you. You may want to go back over the material, discuss it with a friend or just sit with it for awhile. The first book I read on consciousness, I reread seven times and I am still digesting its contents.

☐ Take care of your **Liver**. Organic Dandelion root tea and diluted lemon water are excellent for the liver. Add them to your diet.

☐ **Nourish** yourself.

☐ Rework the **contents of your consciousness** until you achieve the level of function and contentment you want. When discontent, look inside yourself first to see if a shift of perception changes how you feel. We will explore new and exciting ways of shifting perception.

☐ Stay close to your growing **edges**. If you notice that you are experiencing an unhealthy amount of depression then look to where you have moved away from your personal direction for growth. **You only need to move 1\4 of an inch in the right direction to start feeling better.**

☐ Use an essential oil of your choice when studying to **anchor** (purposely connect something less tangible like information with something more tangible like a specific scent) **your new knowledge.** When you want to recall experiences and information gained from the book, smell the oil to help stimulate your recall.

☐ The seasons affect our well being. Working with the seasons develops a natural order to our rituals of well being. Using this natural order is a great advantage. Keep a journal of the seasons so you can reflect on their influence on you over the years.

☐ We live in two worlds simultaneously. One is our everyday world and how we identify ourselves. The other is the hidden world and parts we don't identify with. To achieve a solid sense of well being it is essential to understand both worlds. We call one world our **Ordinary World** and the other world our **Dream World**.

☐ There are three **active forces** that govern life. They are Wind (Vata - Ether & Air) that governs movement. Fire (Pitta - Fire & Water) that governs transformations. Water (Kapha - Earth & Water) which governs growth and stability. All individuals are born with varying blends of all three. By understanding our unique blend we are in a better position to make more informed decisions. I have replaced the words vata, pitta, kapha with the English words wind, fire and water.

☐ Herbs are a special category of plants that help us maintain higher levels of health. They offer us an ecologically sound system of health care. Herbs are a renewable resource and many of them can be grown locally.

☐ Sad but true, most people's lives are a series of interruptions and disruptions. How we choose to view and utilize disruptions has a pronounced effect on our level of wellness.

☐ A sense of personal growth is essential to a feeling of well being. There are many effective methods to choose from that encourage growth.

☐ We need support, knowledge and guidance to achieve and maintain a high level of wellness.

☐ Constantly remind yourself to **focus on the person** more than the disease.

☐ Gentleness brings greater changes. In working your way through the material in this book, be aware that you will have the season that you are working on again next year and the next etc. Be gentle with yourself!

"Educate not medicate"
Bernard Jensen, a leader in the field of natural medicine.

Section 1
Ayurveda

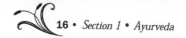
Ayurvedic Constitution

LIFE • LIGHT • LOVE

Air (Vata-Life), Fire (Pitta-Light) and Water (Kapha-Love) are the 3 principles most fundamental to life. They represent, in order, the cosmic urges to movement, transformation and stability (cohesion).

After thirty years of using herbs I feel strongly that it is important to learn the energetics of the tastes and to choose our herbs and foods according to our desired goal. Our goal is to favour the foods and herbs that balance and strengthen our constitution. To know which tastes will get us back into balance when we have taken a learning journey into imbalance. Many diseases can be remedied through interventions that balance the constitution. This knowledge can be used to educate people on health choices and lifestyle decisions. It is truly a wholistic approach that reaches deep into the body and psyche of an individual and offers them wise counsel in every area. This is a remarkable system and I encourage you to study it further if you find it appealing.

I have purposely chosen to use the English names of wind, fire and water.

Western medicine has made a deliberate attempt to separate religion and medicine. Ayurveda sees the two as inseparable. In my practice I did as much or more emotional and spiritual counselling as suggesting herbs and other physical regimes. Disease is usually an opportunity to examine our life a little deeper and see where we may have wandered from our path.

By the end of this section you will be able to:
1) Recognize your own unique Ayurvedic Constitution.
2) Define other's constitutions.
3) Design a program for each constitution.
4) Define what to do to imbalance your constitution.
5) Recognize the four pillars of healing and be sure they are all present when healing.

Do This!

Exercise 5 • *Personal Constitution questionnaire:*

Go through this questionnaire (you may want to photocopy extras first) and check off the choice or choices that best describe you. There might be two for a category, so check off both. The more times you do the questionnaire, you develop a better sense of the three constitutions. It is helpful if you can do the questionnaire with a supportive friend who knows you well.

PHYSICAL

	Wind (Vata)	Fire (Pitta)	Water (Kapha)
Frame (compactness):	☐ thin ☐ irregular	☐ moderate	☐ thick
Bones:	☐ light	☐ medium	☐ heavy
Shoulders:	☐ narrow	☐ medium	☐ broad
Chest:	☐ thin, small ☐ narrow	☐ medium	☐ broad, ☐ well developed
Body weight:	☐ low, thin ☐ difficult to gain weight	☐ moderate ☐ hard to gain weight	☐ heavy, ☐ gains weight easily
Skin:	☐ dry, cold ☐ brownish	☐ oily, warm ☐ pink	☐ oily, cool ☐ white
Head:	☐ narrow	☐ medium	☐ broad
Hair:	☐ dry (dandruff) ☐ kinky, curly ☐ brownish, dull	☐ oily (thin) ☐ blonde, straight ☐ greying, bald	☐ slightly oily ☐ thick, wavy ☐ strong
Teeth:	☐ crooked	☐ gums bleed easily	☐ strong

	Wind:	Fire:	Water:
Lips:	☐ thin, small, dry	☐ med., soft, red	☐ full, smooth
Eyes:	☐ small, active	☐ sharp	☐ large
		☐ penetrating	
	☐ busy	☐ intense, burning	☐ attractive
	☐ dry	☐ bloodshot	☐ watery
Eyebrows:	☐ thin, dry, scaly	☐ moderate	☐ thick
Hands:	☐ small, thin, dry	☐ moderate	☐ large, thick
	☐ cold, rough	☐ warm, pink	☐ oily, cool, firm
Appetite:	☐ variable	☐ excessive	☐ moderate
	☐ low blood sugar	☐ feed me NOW	☐ can go w\o
Hunger every:	☐ 2 hours	☐ 4 hours	☐ 6 hours
Reaction to medicine:	☐ quick	☐ moderate	☐ slow
	☐ low dosage	☐ normal dosage	☐ high dosage
	☐ side effects	☐ sensitive to	☐ effects slow
	☐ nervous reactions	aspirin	
Thirst:	☐ variable	☐ excessive	☐ scanty
Elimination stool: movement:	☐ dry, hard	☐ soft, oily	☐ thick, oily
	☐ constipated	☐ loose	☐ slow
	☐ 1 a day, maybe	☐ 2 to 3 a day	☐ 1 a day
Urination:	☐ scanty, difficult	☐ profuse, yellow	☐ moderate
	☐ colourless	☐ hot, strong odour	☐ milky
Sweat:	☐ rarely, dry	☐ lots, strong odour	☐ moderate
Menstruation:	☐ scanty, painful	☐ moderate to heavy	☐ regular
	☐ cramps, irregular		

	Wind:	Fire:	Water:
Physical activity:	☐ very busy, manic	☐ moderate	☐ little
Endurance:	☐ low	☐ moderate	☐ lots

Sleep:	☐ restless
	☐ dead tired
	  or insomnia
		☐ little
		  but sound
			☐ deep
			☐ prolonged

Climate preference:	☐ warm, wet	☐ cold	☐ warm, dry
Diseases:	☐ neurological ☐ M.S., Parkinson ☐ neurosis ☐ depression ☐ anxiety ☐ pain	☐ bleeding ☐ haemorrhage ☐ inflammation ☐ infections ☐ fever ulcers	☐ common cold ☐ excess mucus ☐ respiratory ☐ swelling
Pulse:	Left wrist~women	Right wrist~men	
	☐ rapid, irregular ☐ snake (slithers)	☐ moderate ☐ frog (hops)	☐ slow, full ☐ swan (glides)
Felt strongest under:	☐ index finger	☐ middle	☐ ring

(Take your pulse early in the morning, on an empty stomach,
after a bowel movement and/or urination.)

Totals: _____   _____   _____

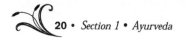

MENTAL\EMOTIONAL

	Wind:	Fire:	Water:
Mind:	☐ restless, active ☐ lively, curious ☐ easily influenced	☐ intense ☐ influential	☐ calm, slow ☐ not easily influenced
Emotions:	☐ fearful, anxious	☐ impatient, angry ☐ jealous ☐ warm ☐ enjoys strong contact	☐ indifferent ☐ love, affection
Beliefs:	☐ changeable	☐ fanatical ˌ	☐ steady
Memory:	☐ recent, good ☐ long term, poor	☐ sharp ☐ selective	☐ slow but prolonged
Dreams:	☐ fearful, flying ☐ running away	☐ colourful ☐ intense ☐ combative	☐ romantic ☐ watery
Speech:	☐ quick, talkative	☐ sharp, convincing	☐ slow, definite

Money:	☐ poor, spends
	   on anything
		☐ moderate, spends
		   on quality
			☐ rich, spends
			   on food

Quality:	☐ inventive	☐ engineer	☐ manager

Sex drive:	☐ mental
	   more in the mind
		☐ active
		   easily aroused
			☐ moderate
			   slow to arouse,
			   but stays aroused

Occupied path:	☐ auditory	☐ visual	☐ proprioceptive
Remembers:	☐ sound	☐ sight	☐ feeling
Reaction:	☐ fear	☐ anger	☐ tension
Totals:	_____	_____	_____

Example: A robber comes into a bank and pulls out a gun and tells everyone to stick up their hands. What do you do ?

a) put up your hands immediately and start praying ?

b) put your hands up slowly while calculating how you can trick the robber and make him pay for interrupting your banking ?

c) walk out in disbelief, realize a block later what is happening and call the police.

Answers:

a) Wind   b) Fire   c) Water

Please redo this questionnaire 2 or 3 times. Do it with a friend who knows you well and can help fill in any holes. Think about the different aspects for a couple of months and observe yourself. Most people are a mixed constitution, often with one predominant constitution.

I find the knowledge I use and learn from Ayurveda to be vitally important to me personally and professionally. It is a fascinating and rewarding study. Good Health!

> ## Do This!
> ### Exercise 6 • *Observing Constitutions*
> Spend a few days in a public place, where you can observe people. Go through each part of the questionnaire and pick out the different constitutions. Example: Lips. Do they have small, thin, dry lips? Or medium, soft, red lips? Or full, firm and smooth? Think about the effect of wind, fire and water and its presence or absence in what you observe.

What Constitution Am I?

You have done the questionnaire and you are still wondering what constitution you are?

WIND

- ☐ You love to be busy.
- ☐ You often have long lists of what you want to get done.
- ☐ You enjoy talking.
- ☐ Your hair is dry and somewhat curly.
- ☐ You have cold feet and hands.
- ☐ Your body is slender.
- ☐ You sometimes suffer from gas or constipation.
- ☐ You often experience fear (be honest).

FIRE

- ☐ You are usually warm.
- ☐ You have warm hands and feet.
- ☐ You hate waiting in lines and are sometimes impatient.
- ☐ Your hair is fine, straight and often oily.
- ☐ You go to the bathroom frequently.
- ☐ You love challenges and even a good fight once in awhile.
- ☐ You particularly enjoy the visual world and often dream in colour.
- ☐ You often experience anger, frustration and impatience (be honest).

WATER

- ☐ You have fairly thick, wavy and oily hair.
- ☐ You are often cool and you like to be warm.
- ☐ You gain weight easily and it is difficult to lose.
- ☐ You like to have lots of food in the cupboards.
- ☐ You enjoy and need at least eight hours of sleep.
- ☐ You tend to avoid stress when possible.
- ☐ You think that most exercise is a waste of time and energy (be honest).

Mixed Constitutions:

Many of us are mixed constitutions. I have a Fire\Water body with a Fire\Wind mind. Fire is the predominant element in my make-up and I need to keep it in balance to feel good. When I first discovered Ayurveda I was living on yoghurt and suffering from a constant burning in my stomach. Sour is the most heating taste and by cutting back, my symptoms quickly disappeared.

My wife Sandy has a Water\Fire body with a predominantly Fire mind. She grew up in the Pacific Northwest and never realized how badly the damp cold affected her until we took a seven week break in the tropics. She especially loved the dry heat and many of her symptoms disappeared. Her fire mind is pro-active, unfortunately her Water body doesn't always want to follow. She feels best when she gets lots of exercise and she is in a warm climate.

Be patient (if you don't have too much fire) and you will get to know your constitution as you begin to understand the workings of Ayurvedic philosophy. The best thing to do when you are of a mixed constitution is to strengthen and build the missing dosha. If you are fire\water then you would encourage the development of air.

Three Functional Levels of Constitutions

WIND:

Harmonious: lots of energy, adaptable, quick thinking and good understanding, communicable, enthusiastic, optimistic, good healing power, ability to make changes easily.

Disturbed: hyperactive, unstable, poor decision making, restless, talks a lot, anxious, jumpy nerves, superficial, empty enthusiasm.

Darkened: depressed, filled with fear, drug addiction, self-destructive, dishonest, mentally challenged, suicidal.

FIRE:

Harmonious: good perception, sharp intelligence, clarity, enlightened, compassionate, inter-dependent, warm, friendly, brave, excellent guide, strong leadership ability.

Disturbed: controlling, domineering, forces will, manipulative, prone to anger, careless, false pride, impulsive, quick to criticize, ambitious.

Darkened: full of hate, resentful, destructive, criminal tendencies, attracted to the underworld, possible drug dealer.

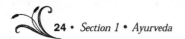

WATER:

Harmonious: compassionate, able to forgive, reliable, nurturing, loving, supportive, devotional, patient, secure, strong faith.

Disturbed: need to control, attachment, greed, materialistic, comfort seeking, insecure, needy, needs luxury.

Darkened: lethargic, lazy, slothful, crude, confused, insensitive, possible thief.

Symptoms of Disturbed Constitutions

	Wind	Fire	Water
Pain:	most intense, tearing, variable, migratory, biting	medium, hot	least, heavy, dull
Fever:	mild, variable, restless	high, sweating, irritable	low, constant
Discharges:	gas, noisy	blood, pus, bile	mucus, watery
Stomach:	irregular appetite, gas	extreme appetite, sour regurgitation, burning, ulcers	slow digestion
Liver & Gall Bladder:	irregular activity	over active, inflamed, gall stones	enlarged, under active.
Faeces:	constipation, difficult, pain, dry, little	frequent, hot, strong odour	slow, large mucus, itching
Urine:	scanty, difficult, colourless	profuse, frequent, hot, yellow, turbid, strong	profuse, white infrequently
Sweat:	scanty, variable	profuse, hot	modest, constant
Mental:	fear, insomnia, apathy	restless, violence	lethargy lacks desire

	Wind	Fire	Water
Time:	dawn, dusk	noon, midnight	mid-morning mid-afternoon
Season:	fall, early winter	late spring, summer	winter, early spring
Disturbs:	wind, cold, dryness	heat, humidity	dampness, cold

How to keep your Constitution in Balance

Following are some suggestions for keeping your constitution in balance when needed. I find it has improved my health, understanding what upsets my constitution and what strengthens it. Being human I still find myself doing things that challenge my constitution but I usually do it with awareness and suffer less than I would have in the past.

I thoroughly enjoy the knowledge that I have gained and I am continually amazed at its accuracy. As you begin to understand yourself and others better, you may develop more understanding and compassion. By being clearer about your expectations of others your relationships may improve.

WIND: Predominant emotion is fear (takes stress and holds onto it)
- ☐ Be regular and practice routine.
- ☐ Start with one project or activity and work on one thing at a time.
- ☐ Get up at the same time every day.
- ☐ Take a hot bath every afternoon.
- ☐ Have a gentle soothing massage with warm oil when stressed.
- ☐ Keep your mind busy, active and happy.
- ☐ Eat small meals frequently:
    - Eat a nourishing diet of sweet, oily, sour & salty edibles.
    - Eat hot, oily, cooked food (root vegetables are excellent).
    - Grains in general are beneficial. Millet is particularly good.
    - Add yoghurt to your diet.
    - Use aromatic herbs.
    - Eat in a relaxed environment.
    - Avoid eating dry foods.

- ☐ Exercise with yoga or tai chi.
- ☐ Surround yourself with less concentrated colours like yellow, orange and pastels.
- ☐ Use alcohol based medicinal preparations like tinctures
- ☐ For those suffering from excess wind: Administer medicated oil enemas. Corrective oily enema is considered the best.

FIRE: Predominant emotion is anger (takes stress and throws it back)

- ☐ Keep pleasant company and environment.
- ☐ Take cold baths or showers.
- ☐ Stay in a cool atmosphere.
- ☐ Administer mild laxatives.
- ☐ Avoid sleeping during the day.
- ☐ Participate in amusement, enjoy music and singing.
- ☐ Food: Favour sweet, bitter and astringent tastes.
  Eat cool salads and other raw foods.
  Eat sufficient quantities.
  Avoid fried foods.
  Avoid excessively pungent spices like cayenne.
  Use ghee (clarified butter) regularly.
  Avoid excess sour foods like tomatoes, yoghurt or wine.
- ☐ Exercise should be cooling like swimming. Avoid competitive sports.
- ☐ For those suffering from excess fire:
  Strong laxatives are considered the best.

WATER: Predominant emotion is complacency (ignores stress)

- ☐ Fast.
- ☐ Exercise.
- ☐ Sleep less.
- ☐ Food: Favour pungent, astringent & bitter tastes.
  Eat dry, non-fatty foods.
  Use stimulating spices like cayenne, ginger and garlic.
  Eat less.
  Avoid fattening foods.
  Use moderate amounts of honey.
- ☐ Have a dry stimulating massage regularly.
- ☐ Use emetics to induce vomiting if lungs become overly congested.
- ☐ Exercise is considered the best for water constitutions.

How to Imbalance Your Constitution
WIND:

- ☐ Fast often.
- ☐ Worry a lot.
- ☐ Never sit down to eat.
- ☐ Stay up late and get up early.
- ☐ Forget about routines.
- ☐ Move around a lot in cars, planes, trains and automobiles.
- ☐ Jog or bounce on a rebounder.
- ☐ Hang out in dry, cold and busy places.
- ☐ Drink lots of coffee.

FIRE:

- ☐ Get drunk a lot.
- ☐ Indulge in hot spices.
- ☐ Involve yourself in frustrating activities.
- ☐ Eat plenty of tomatoes, chillies, raw onions, and sour foods like yoghurt.
- ☐ Add lots of red meat and salted fish to your diet.
- ☐ Snack often on highly salted foods.
- ☐ Exercise at noon in the sun.
- ☐ Over dress.
- ☐ Sleep with the window closed and the heat up.
- ☐ Hang out in hot, stale and violent places.

WATER:

- ☐ Get plenty of sleep during the day.
- ☐ Enjoy fatty foods with lots of extra oil.
- ☐ Eat often and as much as possible especially beer and potato chips.
- ☐ Deny your creativity.
- ☐ Lie around and feel sorry for yourself.
- ☐ Hang-out in cold, dull and wet places.
- ☐ Eat at least one big helping of ice cream or cheese cake every day.
- ☐ Avoid exercise.

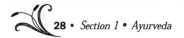

The Four Pillars to Treatment:

In Ayurvedic practice these four components need to be in place if one is going to have a chance of being successful. I have had to counsel clients that they needed an attendent for example.

Herbal Counsellor

Has theoretical knowledge, practical experience, skill, compassion, strong character.

Herbs

Abundantly available. Easily applied. Useful in a variety ways. High quality.

Attendant

Must be knowledgable in nursing skills, affectionate and clean.

Patient

Needs to have clear recollection, discipline with instructions, commitment, the ability to describe ailments and changes.

CONGESTION & BIO-FIRE

In this section we will explore congestion from an Ayurvedic viewpoint. How it is created and what is its affect on each of the constitutions? How to recognize it and remove it. You will learn how to prevent it by building a strong bio-fire.

By the end of this section you will be able to:
1) Know how to recognize congestion in each constitution and what steps to take to relieve it.
2) Recognize good bio-fire by the colour of the nail beds.
3) Prevent congestion by building strong bio-fire (digestion).

CONGESTION (AMA)
- ☐ Accumulation of toxins, waste materials and indigestible food consisting largely of mucoid accretions.
- ☐ Opposite of Bio-Fire.
- ☐ Psychologically, emotional congestion arises from holding onto negative emotions.
- ☐ Indigestible experiences become toxic like indigestible food. We may need help breaking them down into digestible experiences.

Qualities: ☐ Heavy   ☐ Cloudy   ☐ Dense   ☐ Strong odour
              ☐ Cold   ☐ Slimy   ☐ Impure

Symptoms: ☐ Loss of taste and appetite.   ☐ Indigestion.
            ☐ Coated tongue.   ☐ Bad breath.
            ☐ Loss of strength.   ☐ Heaviness and lethargy.
            ☐ Obstruction of channels   ☐ Accumulation of
              and vessels.   waste materials.

            ☐ Bad odour of body,   ☐ Lack of attention.
              urine and faeces.
            ☐ Loss of clarity.   ☐ Depression.
            ☐ Irritability.   ☐ Deep, heavy or dull pulse.

Ama is the root of a weak auto-immune system, which can lead to colds, fevers, flus and chronic diseases e.g. allergies, hayfever, asthma, arthritis and cancer. Severe AMA is rare and presents a difficult condition.

Gently Eliminate Congestion (Ama) first (if obvious) before treating the Constitution!

☐ Use bitter tasting herbs and foods. Bitter separates the congesting materials lodged in the tissues and organs. Stimulates catabolism breaking down foreign material.

☐ Use pungent tasting herbs and foods. Pungent burns up and eradicates congestion.

☐ Take bitter first to halt the development and pungent to strengthen the Bio-Fire. Bio-Fire promotes the consumption of congestion and prevents it from returning.

☐ Congestion makes us feel heavy. I recommend cleansing, using herbs and foods of a light nature and exercising more.

Balancing the Constitutions

Pacify the constitution disturbed (likely Wind). Wind brings Fire and Water into line. Treat Wind with rest, meditation, warmth and massage.

We treat congestion first **if present**. **Sama** means there is **Ama** interfering with the function of the element. **Nirama** means there is no Ama involved. Severe AMA is rare and excess cleansing disturbs the body and the mind.

WIND:

SAMA	NIRAMA
With Congestion:	Without Congestion:
(Deficient Wind)	(Excess Wind)
constipation	regular, once a day
foul breath and faeces	moderate smell
abdominal pain and distention	a little distention
aggravated by touch	soothed by touch
gas and cramping	none
coated tongue-low appetite	dry tongue-good appetite
heaviness	light feeling
weakness-fatigue	more energy
slow pulse	rapid pulse
aggravated by cloudy weather	not aggravated

Treatment:

Cleanse:
short fast - three days

Tone:
Nutrition

FIRE:

SAMA
With Congestion:
(Deficient Fire)

NIRAMA
Without Congestion:
(Excess Fire)

loss of appetite	excess appetite
little thirst	excess thirst
yellow tongue coating	red, inflamed, no coating
urine, faeces mucus-yellow green	same-red or clear
heaviness in the stomach	stomach feels empty
thick bilious vomiting	
bad breath	breath normal
bitter or sour taste in the mouth	
mild burning sensations	strong burning sensations
skin rash	hot flashes, dizziness
cloudy perceptions	sharp perceptions
aggravated by cold	aggravated by heat

Treatment:

Cleanse:
fast five to seven days,
bitter, pungent and stimulant herbs

To cool and tone:
Sweet and bitter foods
and herbs

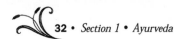

WATER:

Sama	Nirama
With Congestion:	Without Congestion:
(Deficient Water)	(Excess Water)

mucus cloudy sticky or thick	watery or frothy mucus
blocks throat and coats tongue	tongue clear
sour or salty taste in the mouth	sweet taste
congestion and tightness in chest	no congestion
difficulty breathing	breathing easy
mucus in stool and urine	none
low appetite	normal
heaviness, dull aching	
generalized pain, fatigue	

Cleanse: Tone:
fast seven to ten days   Pungent and Sweet taste.
take pungent and bitter herbs
expectorants, stimulants and decongestants

BIO-FIRE (AGNI)

- ☐ Biological processes of digestion, metabolism and catabolism.
- ☐ Gastric secretions.
- ☐ Acidic in nature.
- ☐ Present in every tissue and cell.
- ☐ Supports the nutrition of every cell and tissue.
- ☐ Maintains the auto immune function.
- ☐ Destroys microorganisms, foreign bacteria and toxins in the small and large intestines and stomach.
- ☐ Affects intelligence, understanding, perception and comprehension.
- ☐ Gives colour to the skin.
- ☐ Ruler of the enzyme system.

Impaired Bio-Fire:

- ☐ Lowered resistance to disease and immune function.
- ☐ Food particles remain indigestible and unabsorbed, clogging the intestines, capillaries and blood vessels. They develop into toxins that are absorbed into the blood and enter general circulation. They settle in weak areas in the body and develop into chronic conditions like arthritis, diabetes and heart disease.

Finger nails:
- ❏ Pink and rosy = good bio-fire
- ❏ Pale and dull = poor bio-fire

AYURVEDIC GUIDELINES

❏ Use Ayurveda as a paradigm for processing the mass of new information avaliable today and organizing it for your future use.

❏ Remember that "like increases like". Under certain circumstances, "like cures like" but always "like increases like", by the principle of its effect (resonance - vibration).

❏ At the junction of the seasons, air, fire and water are realigning themselves. Pay closer attention to your constitution and its needs at these times. The stronger the seasonal change the greater the effect.

❏ When healing with diet, choose tastes and temperature antagonistic to principle in excess. e.g. To reduce excess Fire eat more bitter tasting and cooler food like salads. Watch for foods that may be aggravating your condition or constitution and eliminate or reduce depending on the severity of the condition. Build up your power of digestion with short fasts, exercise and bitter taste. Lemon water is extremely helpful with meals.

❏ Honour your own and everyone's uniqueness. Each person has a unique connection to the universe.

❏ Disease may be the result of improper adaption to change. Use dreambody tools to process your changes when ill or preferably before you get ill. Take time to process your feelings when making any major changes. Your body will appreciate and reward you.

❏ Either decide that something will be good for you, or avoid it.

❏ Build when the person is weak. Purify when the disease is weak and the person is strong. Too much purification disturbs wind. Relax and enjoy your life without excessive concern for your well being when you are feeling good.

- ☐ Learn to listen to your senses more often. When you are not listening to your five senses, you gather false information and develop false desires. When feeling confused use all your senses to pick up sensory-grounded information around you.

- ☐ See what you are seeing. Hear what you are hearing. Sense what your body is feeling. Pay attention to any movements you are making. Smell what you are smelling and taste what you are tasting.

- ☐ Obstructions on the path of your desires and obstacles to your escape routes from pain upset the balance of your constitution.

Taste

In this section we begin to explore the subjective realm of knowledge by taking you on a personal journey through the land of the six tastes. We begin to use more of our body and psyche for learning. It is important to participate to the best of your abilities and stretch your imagination into the many paths that we walk on this journey. By taking the time to explore each of the areas that I ask you about you will be expanding your experience and you may or may not be surprised at what may surface.

By the end of this section you will be able to:
1) Use the understanding of the six qualities and the six tastes to make informed decisions on the right interventions to help yourself or someone else.
2) Explore the nine paths of the journey.
3) Know what each of the tastes do for you.

TASTE

Taste is largely social and has a powerful social element. Most special gatherings and events are celebrated with food. Meal times bring families together where they learn many of the family patterns. Tasting is probably our main source of pleasure. Our goal is to increase and deepen that pleasure by increasing your experience and knowledge of the different tastes. A person who has taste is someone who has eaten heartily of life and developed a sense of the sublime and the gross.

—Diane Ackerman

Taste according to Ayurveda:
- ❏ is the essence of the plant.
- ❏ communicates feelings.
- ❏ directly affects the nervous system awakening the mind and senses.
- ❏ awakens Bio-Fire, enhancing our power of digestion.
- ❏ sets our digestive fluids in motion.

Lack of taste leads to:
- ❏ low Bio-Fire.
- ❏ excess Congestion.

To improve Bio-Fire and eliminate disease it is necessary to improve our sense of taste. If the tongue is heavily coated consider a short fast. Increase your consumption of zinc. Get more exercise.

POST DIGESTIVE EFFECT (Vipaka):
The effect that a taste has after it has been digested.
- ❏ Sweet\Salty = Sweet
- ❏ Sour =Sour
- ❏ Bitter\Astringent\ Pungent = Pungent

Digestion
1st. Stage **(Water)** - Mouth and Stomach
- ❏ Moistening
- ❏ Sweet

2nd. Stage **(Fire)** - Stomach and Small Intestine
- ❏ Heating
- ❏ Sour

3rd. Stage **(Wind)** - Colon
- ❏ Drying
- ❏ Pungent

TASTE EXERCISE #7

☐ Expanding awareness of the tastes and linking them to the different paths. Get at least one representative of the various tastes.

☐ Set aside enough time to enjoy and thoroughly experience the tastes.

☐ These six tastes are a fundamental building block of ayurveda and herbalism.

☐ Be sure to let each taste touch every part of your tongue. We taste sweet things with the tip, bitter at the back, sour on both sides and salty things spread over the surface of our tongue.

☐ Pungent and astringent are more of a sensation than a taste.

☐ Our taste buds detect:
> Sweet in 1 part to 200.
> Salt is detected in 1 in 400.
> Sour is 1 in 130,000.
> Bitter is 1 in 2,000,000 parts.

☐ We need moistness to taste.

Healing Journey Taste Class (Example)

Giant Fir trees dotted the parking lot. The air was cold and crisp. You could smell the sea. There was a feeling of expectant anticipation. These students were my researchers. We were exploring new alchemical modes of awareness. We unpacked our equipment and headed for the beach. The leaves crunched under our feet. The sun was shining but the wind had a cold bite to it. We snuggled together for warmth.

The first taste we explored was sweet. I passed around some medjool dates and each student began their experiment. Some plunged the whole date in their mouth while others nibbled at the edges. Soon eyes were closing as students absorbed their attention into the sweetness. When I teach I usually do the exercises with my students so I will be in the experience with them. I bit off about half. The sweetness was intense and I allowed my taste buds to indulge in the orgy of sweetness. After sufficient time to explore sweetness in all the paths we came back together to share.

Some students found the sweetness thick, heavy and sticky. All of us noted the lasting quality of the taste. We felt a sense of sustained energy especially with the natural sugars of the date. Most felt it satisfying. We tried white sugar later and found it to have an empty quality. In the relationship path some found sweetness to be little acts of kindness. While others thought of sexual intimacy. Some felt their relationships provided the sweetness they needed while others sensed a lack and needed more. One student later divorced her husband. These experiences can often tap into areas of denial or unawareness. In the world path students thought of sweetness as a good job, others as a happy home and for some freedom gave them that sense of sweetness. For me it was doing the work I love in a place I love to be. Spiritually sweetness was most represented by contentment.

Next we did salt. I handed out some fantastic kelp powder harvested, processed and distributed by my friend Ryan Drum. I love salt. The moment I put it in my mouth I felt good. I felt it pulled together all the fibres of my being. I could smell the salt in the air and feel the ocean in my cells. Visually it was crystalline. I remembered pictures of processing sea water through natural solar evaporation.

I thought about all the different mineral salts. I crave salt. It is my addiction and when I am stressed-out I crave salted pumpkin seeds before any other taste. Salt as a movement was drawing me into a focused and still meditation posture. In relationship I thought of licking the salty tears of my lover. Also the power of attraction that draws souls to each other. The sound was clear, crisp and metallic like a high pitched symbol. In my world it is scuba diving. I feel totally satisfied after a good dive. Spiritually I find it centering and usually crave it more when I am in transition and there is a certain degree of chaos around.

Some of the students found the salty taste too intense. The experiences in the group were more polarized around salt than sweet.

Next we did pungent. I used fresh Ginger root for the pungent taste. When we compared notes we found more of a consensus with this taste. We all found it stimulating but not lasting like sweet. In relationships it was passion or conflict. Many of us felt that a certain amount of conflict was necessary in a healthy relationship. If everyone is thinking the same thing, then someone isn't thinking. Pungent definitely encouraged more movement than sweet and salty. There was a sense that pungent could be nicely moderated with the addition of sweet. And of course sweet could be motivated with a little addition of pungent. In the world pungent was more associated with action. Pungent feelings exist closer to the edges of the things we want to do but are afraid of trying. The closer we move to the edge of doing them, the more our life heats up. Pungent is heating. Spiritually it was spirited action.

Next I passed around slices of lemon. Another intense taste. I love lemons. I think they are one of the magic foods. I feel that everyone would benefit by discovering their magic foods. When they need a little magic in their life they can use them. Most of the students nibbled at the lemon. Almost everyone found it cleansing. Lemon cleans your mouth of the other tastes and leaves your tongue feeling clean. Sour was more complex, like salt, and brought out more differences in the students' response to it. This is why I encourage you to establish your own relationship to the tastes and not totally rely on some external system to tell you what they do for you.

Astringent was more of an experience than a taste. It was definitely contracting in all the paths. Bitter was surprising. We found it to be extremely centering and long lasting. Almost all agreed that a certain degree of bitter was beneficial in every path.

I hope you get a sense from this example of what I am asking you to do. I still use some of the insights that I learned on that day when I experience the different qualities of the tastes in my life and how they relate to the different paths.

Do This!

Exercise 7 • *The Six Tastes and the Nine Paths*

Do each taste separately and answer the questions below for each taste.

First smell it. Next place a small amount in your mouth and close your eyes. Allow the taste to penetrate you. Meditate on it for at least 5 minutes. You might want to try moving like it. Now answer the following questions.

SWEET: preferably use a medjool date. Another date will do. You can try other sweets to increase your knowledge of sweet. In one group we tried white sugar. Very revealing.

BITTER: Gentian, Dandelion, Endive etc.

SOUR: Lemon, Vitamin C etc.

SALTY: Salt, Kelp etc.

PUNGENT: Ginger, Garlic, Elecampane etc.

ASTRINGENT: Black tea, Blackberry leaf, Oak bark etc.

* What kind of visions does this taste stimulate?

* What kind of sound do you associate with it?

* What feeling or body sensation does it evoke?

* How would you imagine it moving?

* How would it manifest in your personal relationships?

* What kind of work would fit this taste?

* How do you imagine this flavour in your community?

* How would this taste manifest in the spirit?

* Are you attracted or repulsed by this taste?

* Do you feel you need more or less of this taste?

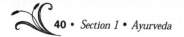

The Six Tastes according to Ayurveda

- means this taste reduces   + means this taste increases

SWEET

Wind\Fire- Water+

Elements: Earth and Water
Qualities: Heavy\wet\cooling
Post Digestive Effect (Vipaka): Sweet

Body Effects:
- ☐ Promotes the growth of all bodily tissues
- ☐ Creates strength and longevity
- ☐ Soothing to the mind and the five senses
- ☐ Increases semen
- ☐ Gives contentment
- ☐ Rebuilds essential energy

Properties:
- ☐ Rebuilds essential energy
- ☐ Rejuvenating
- ☐ Nutritive tonic
- ☐ Demulcent and Emollient

Excess: Obesity, laziness, excessive sleep, heaviness, loss of appetite, weak digestion, abdominal distention, swelling of lymph, aggravates Water

Examples: Licorice, Marshmallow, Slippery elm, Roasted roots, Maple bark, Maple syrup, Licorice Fern root and Raw sugar

Emotions:
- ☐ Lack - Unfulfilled longing
- ☐ Sufficient - Satisfaction

A person may have an unnatural craving for sweets if they are experiencing an excess of frustration and lack of satisfaction. If they learn to use the flow paradigm to regulate their life in a way that increases the amount of satisfaction they may crave less sweets.

BITTER

Wind+ Fire\Water-

Elements: Wind and Ether
Qualities: Cold\light\dry
Post Digestive Effect (Vipaka): Pungent

Body Effects:
- ☐ Restores sense of taste
- ☐ Helps reduce tumours
- ☐ Helps scrape away fat

- ☐ Cleansing to blood and all tissues
- ☐ Enkindles the digestive fire
- ☐ Drains and dries the tissues

Properties:
- ☐ Anti-inflammatory
- ☐ Germicidal

- ☐ Antibacterial
- ☐ Febrifuge

Excess: Wasting away of all tissues, produces roughness, weakening, emancipating, dizziness, dryness (mouth), aggravates Wind.

Examples: Dandelion, Oregon grape root, Goldenseal, Gentian and Endive.

Emotions:
- ☐ Excess - Grief

- ☐ Sufficient - Joy

I had a client who had spent a number of years in a concentration camp. He was a wind constitution. He was very attracted to bitter dandelion greens. He felt that they kept him alive. Even though the dandelions were bitter they brought him a lot of joy.

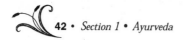

SOUR:

Fire\Water+ Wind-

> **Elements**: Earth and Fire
> **Qualities**: Hot\wet\light
> **Post Digestive Effect (Vipaka)**: Sour

Qualities:
- ☐ Promotes digestion
- ☐ Nourishing to all tissues except reproductive
- ☐ Promotes metabolism and circulation
- ☐ Increases appetite
- ☐ Awakens the mind
- ☐ Gives firmness to the senses
- ☐ Promotes salivation, aids swallowing moistening and digestion of food
- ☐ Drains the liver

Properties:
- ☐ Carminative
- ☐ Stimulant

Excess: Teeth sensitive, causes thirst, blinking of the eyes, aggravates Fire, causing a build up of toxins in the blood.

Examples: Hawthorn berries, Lemons, Rose hips, Sorrel, Alcohol & Fermentation.

Emotions:
- ☐ Excess - Envy
- ☐ Sufficient- Contentment

There was a period of time in my life when I ate a lot of sour. I experienced very little contentment and my fire was constantly in excess. I was involved in a sour relationship at the time. That relationship was dissolved and new ones were begun. I now experience more contentment and less envy. When I am suffering from excess envy I take it as a clue to a possible new direction that I may want to go.

PUNGENT

Wind\Fire+ Water-

Elements: Wind and Fire
Qualities: Hot\dry\light
Post Digestive Effect (Vipaka): Pungent

Body Effects:
- ☐ Stimulating: increasing circulation and bodily functions
- ☐ Removes waste material
- ☐ Dispersing and moving effect
- ☐ Increases appetite and promotes digestion
- ☐ Intensifies and prolongs the effects of the other herbs.

Properties:
- ☐ Diaphoretic - skin
- ☐ Expectorant - lungs
- ☐ Vermicide - digestive tract

Excess: Gives burning sensations, tremors, stabbing pains, weariness and dizziness.

Examples: Cayenne, Cinnamon, Ginger, Garlic (volatile oils), Propolis and Myrrh (resins)

Emotions:
- ☐ Excess - Anger
- ☐ Sufficient - Excitement

I often think of people as different herbs. One student I had was very pungent like Cayenne. Others found her difficult to take regularly or in large doses. I encouraged her to become more like Ginger. Anger is sometimes connected to a sense of loss. Figure out what you have lost and agree to let it go or make arrangements to try and get it back. This is more exciting than suffering from excess anger.

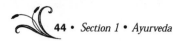

SALTY

Fire\Water+ Wind-

Elements: Water and Fire
Qualities: Wet\heavy\hot
Post Digestive Effect (Vipaka): Sweet

Body Effects:
- ☐ Moistens and softens organs.
- ☐ Creates salivation.
- ☐ Gives taste to food
- ☐ Promotes digestion
- ☐ Liquifies congestion
- ☐ Draws herbs to the kidneys

Properties:
- ☐ Sedative
- ☐ Laxative

Excess: Internal bleeding, hyper-acidity, inflammation, gout, aggravates Fire

Examples: Sea salt, Rock salt, Seaweed

Emotions:
- ☐ Excess - Greed
- ☐ Sufficient - Zest

When we have too much greed in our lives we are weighed down by our possessions. Sometimes a give away is just the thing we need to put some zest back in our life. We also need a certain amount of desire to propel us forward.

ASTRINGENT

Wind+ Fire\Water-

Elements: Earth and Wind
Qualaties: Cold\dryheavy
Post Digestive Effect (Vipaka): Pungent

Body Effects:
- ☐ Contracts the muscles helping to raise prolapsed organs
- ☐ Stops sweating
- ☐ Stops diarrhoea
- ☐ Promotes absorption of fluids

Properties:
- ☐ Haemostatic (stops bleeding)
- ☐ Vulnerary
- ☐ Anti-inflammatory

Excess: Drying of the mouth, pain in the heart, constipation, weakens the voice, obstructs paths of circulation, aggravates Wind.

Examples: Plantain, Red raspberry leaves, Ladies' mantle, White oak bark.

Emotions:
- ☐ Excess - Fear
- ☐ Sufficient - Courage

Excess fear is hard on our health. We are constantly on alert. We benefit by exercising our courage sometimes and facing our fears. Fear can cause us to live a constricted life. By facing them and overcoming them slowly our life expands.

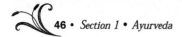

ENERGETICS (VIRYA)

The immediate effect that a taste has on the body.

Heating - pungent\sour\salty
- ☐ Pungent - Ginger
- ☐ Sour - Lemon
- ☐ Salty - Salt

Cooling - bitter\astringent\sweet
- ☐ Bitter - Gentian
- ☐ Astringent - White oak bark
- ☐ Sweet - Licorice.

TASTES & ORGANS

Excess sweet disturbs the spleen.
Excess pungent disturbs the lungs.
Excess bitter disturbs the heart.

Excess salty disturbs the kidneys.
Excess sour disturbs the liver.
Excess astringent disturbs the colon.

QUALITIES

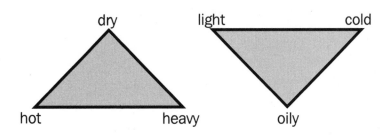

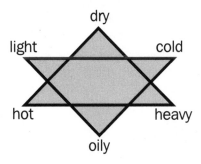

TASTES
(that reduce)

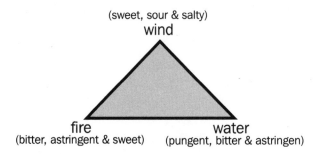

(sweet, sour & salty)
wind

fire
(bitter, astringent & sweet)

water
(pungent, bitter & astringen)

TRI - CONSTITUTIONAL CHART

* Bach Flower Remedies for prominent emotions of each dosha tastes

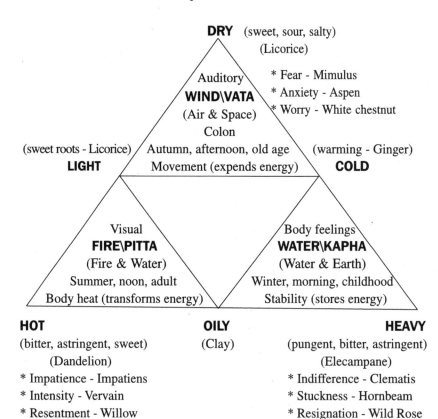

DRY (sweet, sour, salty)
(Licorice)

Auditory
WIND\VATA
(Air & Space)
Colon

* Fear - Mimulus
* Anxiety - Aspen
* Worry - White chestnut

(sweet roots - Licorice)
LIGHT

Autumn, afternoon, old age
Movement (expends energy)

(warming - Ginger)
COLD

Visual
FIRE\PITTA
(Fire & Water)
Summer, noon, adult
Body heat (transforms energy)

Body feelings
WATER\KAPHA
(Water & Earth)
Winter, morning, childhood
Stability (stores energy)

HOT
(bitter, astringent, sweet)
(Dandelion)
* Impatience - Impatiens
* Intensity - Vervain
* Resentment - Willow
* Hate - Holly

OILY
(Clay)

HEAVY
(pungent, bitter, astringent)
(Elecampane)
* Indifference - Clematis
* Stuckness - Hornbeam
* Resignation - Wild Rose

Do This!
Exercise 8

Study this chart! It contains the essence of Ayurveda energetics.
Herbs (in brackets) that reduce/balance the dosha/quality e.g.
ginger warms cold, bitter cools hot, clay reduces oily. Includes time
of day, time of life and season when dosha is most active. Also most
commonly occupied pathway e.g. Fire - Visual.

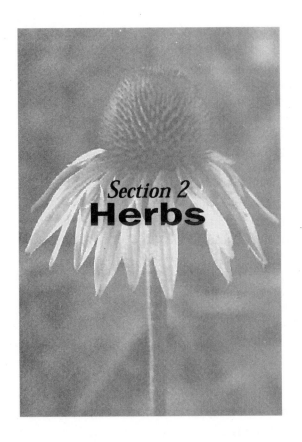

Section 2
Herbs

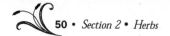

Herbal Preparations
& Medicine Making

We are as much a product of our herbal preparations as they are a product of us. Creating medicines creates a medicine maker. We are all potential medicine makers. I can usually tell when I wake up whether it is going to be a good day for making medicine. Before beginning, I visualize the process in my mind, making notes of the supplies I will need. It is ideal to have a special space set up with all your tools for making medicines, otherwise you can improvise. Sometimes I make tinctures right in the forest where I harvest the herbs.

Medicine making is an art. We can isolate and duplicate all the components of a Stradivarius violin but we cannot reproduce one. Every person, plant, day and moment is unique. Cherish that uniqueness! No two people will make an herbal preparation the same and no one has the final word on what is THE right way.

My definition of an herbalist is **one who has a vital link to Nature and helps others to bond with her.** Making medicines is a process that deepens and potentiates your contact with Nature and her marvellously enchanting ways. Making medicine is a healing process. You needn't be a medicine maker to be an herbalist but it helps to be familiar with the process and certain that the medicines you are using are of the highest quality. I personally encourage you to go through the medicine making process so that you will develop a feeling for the art.

Your Herbal Medicines can only be as
Good as the Quality of the Herbs you Use!

I prefer wildcrafted herbs if they are harvested ecologically. Next are the ones that have been carefully and lovingly cultivated. It is good to talk to your plants and tell them of your INTENT in growing and harvesting them. Choose ones grown with good intent and high standards.

INFUSION: Water Extraction

Standard Infusion: 1 tsp. (5ml) to 1 cup (250ml) of boiling water. Steep 5 to 10 min.

Medium Infusion: 2 tsp to 1 cup

Strong infusion: 4 tsp to 1 cup

> ### Do This!
>
> **Exercise 9** • *Solar Infusion: Sun & Water extraction*
>
> Place some of your favourite herbs (preferrably volatile lvs and flowers) dry or fresh in a clear glass jar with cold water. Leave out in the direct sun for at least 4 hrs., preferably between 10am and 2pm. For added strength you can place your favourite crystal in the jar while it is brewing.

Lunar infusion - to capture the power and magic of a full moon do the same except you will place the jar in the rays of moonlight. Best with fresh picked flowers.

Decoction: Usually used for tough leaves, roots, some berries and barks. Same proportions as infusion except you simmer the herbs for a given time. e.g. Hawthorn berries.

TINCTURE:

Generally the ratio used is 1:5, which means 1 gr. of herb to 5 ml. of menstrum (liquid they are in, usually alcohol). Vodka is good for most tinctures. We then macerate the herb in the menstrum for 10 to 14 days. I strongly recommend leaving them longer. A good time to start it is on the new moon & complete on the full moon. Some people like to use a blender to grind the herbs. I prefer to cut the herb as fine as possible and not blend. Shake the tincture 2 to 3 x a day. When the tincture is ready, strain it through fine cotton or strong cheese cloth and press it by hand. Label it with name, date, quality and batch number.

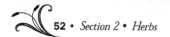

Do This!

Exercise 10 • *Making a Tincture: Alcohol Extraction*

Dried Herb 1:5 Ratio 40% Menstruum

- Purchase yourself a bottle of Vodka.

- Get six ounces of an herb that you use regularly.

- Measure out 30 fluid ounces of Vodka and pour into a large mouth jar.

- Powder, grind or cut up fine the six ounces of herb.

- Now add the herb to the alcohol.

- Put on a tight leak prove lid and seal.

- Label the tincture.

- Leave in a convenient place where you can shake it twice a day. Make sure that all the herb is submerged in the alcohol. Depending on the herb you choose you may need to add a little more Vodka if it all gets absorbed. You want some fluidity and washing motion when you shake it.

- After two weeks minimum (some can be left for months) strain through silk or fine cheese cloth.

- Bottle and label. You now have your own tincture.

- Keep a file card on your procedure and make notes on what you might do differently next time. Experiment with leaving the herbs in different lengths of time for varying strengths.

- Make small batches of as many herbs as you can to gain experience (the best teacher). Use small jars. Practice makes good medicine. Keep clear notes.

FRESH HERB TINCTURE

Ratio:

- determine by weighing amount of fresh herb that fits into jar finely chopped
- measure amount of alcohol needed to cover the herb with 1 inch over top of herb
- divide weight into volume to establish ratio many books suggest a 1:2 Ratio which we find unrealistic for most herbs

Menstruum: % depends on herb

Saturation Tincture: amount of herb that will fit into established amount of menstruum

Glycerine Tincture: 6 parts vegetable glycerine\4 parts water

6 parts vegetable glycerine\3 parts water\1 part alcohol

Use glycerine mix in place of Alcohol

VINEGAR: (Tincture)

Use same instructions as fresh tincture but use apple cider vinegar as menstruum. Buy a high quality organic vinegar. For nutritive herbs like Nettles, Horsetail, Alfalfa or Red Clover you can make a saturation vinegar. Don't worry about proportions, just add as much herb as will fit and still allow the liquid to move around. Make small batches of a lot of different herbs. Experiment!

LINIMENT:

We make these the same way as tinctures.

OIL:

We use a high quality olive or almond oil. If the plant we are using is excessively moist then let this oil sit undisturbed for 2 weeks, check any water. If there is water, then remove the oil from the top with a baster and check again in another week. Important as water will cause the oil to go rancid.

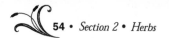

☐ Add some natural preservative like propolis tincture, poplar bud oil or tincture, benzoin tincture or vitamin e oil.

☐ Bottle (dark jars), cap tightly, label and store in a dark cool place.

☐ Make notes of your experiment. You are now becoming an alchemist.

SALVE:

Do This!

Exercise 11 • *Turn your Herbal Oil into a Salve*

Take 1 cup of herbal oil and warm up. Add 1 oz. wt. of grated bees wax a little at a time. Before you add all the wax test the consistency. Take a spoon (that you have had in the freezer) and put a small amount of the mixture on it. Keep adding the wax until you get the desired consistency. Pour into containers and let sit. You can add a drop or 2 of essential oil at this point if you want. Label.

SYRUP:

Make a strong decoction by simmering the herbs to the desired strength. You can sample the brew until it tastes right to you. Add one fourth honey of the total amount you've got. This will usually keep for the duration of a cough or cold. Keep in the fridge. Great for making cough medicine.

HONEY PREPARATION:

Simply add the desired herb to warm honey and let sit in a warm place for a couple of months. Use when needed. Very moist herbs need to be dried first. Great for lung and throat herbs.e.g. fresh evergreen tips from Fir, Hemlock, Balsam, Spruce or Pine.

BOLUS:

Take the powdered herb or herbs and add to melted cocoa butter or coconut oil and mix to pie dough consistency. Shape into middle finger size tubes and wrap in wax paper. Refrigerate until needed. We use these vaginally and rectally (prostate gland).

CLAY:

Mix powdered herb with clay, moisten and apply. Or add herbal infusion or decoction to clay and apply.

CAPSULES:

Do This!

Exercise 12 • *Making your own Capsulated Herbs*

Fill a bowl with the powdered herb or herbs. Remove the small end of the capsule and press the other end into the herbs until it is full then put small end back on. Label, date, store in air tight container in dark place. Use ASAP.

JUICE:

Do This!

Exercise 13 • *Using Fresh Herbs*

Blend the fresh herb of your choice with your favourite juice. When using your juicer add fresh herbs to any juice you are making. Using a wheat grass juicer you can juice the more succulent herbs directly. You can freeze them for future use. Ice cube trays make good proportions. I prefer them fresh.

SOUPS:

Experiment by adding different medicinal herbs when making your soups. e.g. Nettles, Kelp, Dulse, Saffron, Chickweed, Garlic etc. Be creative. A great way to treat the family. Excellent in the Fall (Wind season). Many herbs lend themselves to this method of preparation. Get creative!

SMUDGE:

Burn your favourite herbs to purify and charge the air element in your home, ritual space and aura. My favourites are sweet grass, sage, cedar and wild celery seeds.

WINE:

Make according to your favorite wine recipe.

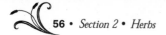

Herbs That Keep You Healthy
How to use herbs to nourish yourself.

HERBAL ALLY

☐ An ally is much greater than a drug.

☐ An Ally is a friend and a power. She can come to your rescue on many levels. She can comfort you at one time and then turn around and challenge you the next time.

☐ Plants are living beings with incredible power and personalities. They want to make contact with people. Most of them are inclusive and want to include us in their lives.

☐ Without plants we wouldn't be breathing or eating.

☐ Herbalism is a living art. The art of living.

☐ The main focus of using the plants is **nourishment.** Eat your weeds!

☐ Healing is what you do between illness events. Eat your weeds!

NOURISH YOUR WHOLE BODY

Stinging Nettle Urtica dioica

Found in the temperate regions of Europe, Britain, Asia, Japan, S. Africa, Australia, Andes and N. America. Indians used it to make cord and fish nets. Used in Britain to make very fine linen. Discontinued because the nettles were too difficult to cultivate.

Uses:

☐ Improves nutrition - high in chlorophyll, iron, magnesium, calcium, phosphate, Vitamin D, silica, sodium, potassium & sulphur.
☐ Good for people who suffer from migraines associated with bilious vomiting.
☐ **Excellent to relieve the symptoms of hayfever & other allergies.**
☐ Purifies the blood and cleanses the lymph.

- Reduces uric acid helping with rheumatism & gout.
- Promotes milk in nursing mothers, Galactagogue.
- Improves digestion - contains secretin, a substance that acts as a stimulus to pancreatic secretion that stimulates the digestive glands of the stomach, intestines, liver & gall bladder.
- Gargling reduces mouth infections, thrush, gingivitis & tonsillitis.
- Use fresh plant to sting an area, usually bothered with rheumatism or arthritis. **I have witnessed it work like a charm.**

Do This!

Exercise 14 • *Nourishing Vinegar*

Make a vinegar, strong infusion or soup using Alfalfa, Horsetail, Kelp and Nettle using instructions from preparation section. Use these herbs regularly as a mineral, vitamin supplement. Add other nutritive herbs as your personal needs dictate.

Dosage: Vinegar - 1 to 2 tsps. in water with meals
            Infusion - 1 to 3 cups a day with meals
            Soup - whenever it appeals to you

NOURISH YOUR BONES, TEETH, CONNECTIVE TISSUE AND LUNGS

Horsetail Equisetum arvense

Uses:

- Recalcification. Osteoporosis.
- Diuretic. The more silica in the body the greater the diuretic effect.
- Healthier fingernails in 15 days.
- Healing fractured bones in 17 days.
- Stimulates rapid recalcification of lung tissue helping with Tuberculosis.
- Teeth. Hardens the enamel. Prevents gum bleeding, gum atrophy & recession. Fights cavities.
- Cancer. Powerful eliminator of organic waste products, particularly urea, uric acid and nicotine. Strengthens connective tissue, the prime barrier set up by the body to ward off the progression of cancer cells and the degenerative process.

☐ Arterial weakness. Clears the arteries and makes them more pliable.
☐ Helps to dissolve kidney stones & clear up urinary tract infections.
☐ Reduces inflammation of the G.I. tract and clears stomach & intestinal catarrh.
☐ Antioxidant.
☐ A natural deodorant.
☐ Prevention & repair of stretch marks.
☐ Promotes healthy collagen. (Check by pinching the skin on the back of your hand to see how it snaps back. Lack of collagen makes it sluggish).

Dosage: Strong infusion - 1/2 to 1 cup 2 to 5 x day with meals
            Tincture - 2 to 5 ml. 2 to 5 x day with meals

NOURISH YOUR THYROID

Kelp

Uses:

☐ Ninety-two different nutritional elements.
☐ Rich source of natural Iodine.
☐ Provides energy and endurance.
☐ Helps relieve nervous tension (excellent for Wind types)
☐ Contains more minerals than land plants. (our land minerals are being carried to the sea by our poor treatment of our soil)
☐ Rich source of potassium.
☐ Helps to pull excess radiation out of the body and to protect against same.
☐ Soothing to the whole gastro-intestinal tract.

Dosage: Powder - 1tsp. 2 to 3 x day with meals
            Caution: **Insist on the highest quality kelp.**

ENCOURAGE THE ASSIMILATION OF YOUR MINERALS & VITAMINS

Apple Cider Vinegar

Uses:

☐ Rich source of readily available potassium.

☐ Helps the body digest food esp. minerals.

☐ Promotes weight loss.

☐ Dissolves unwanted calcium deposits.

☐ Helps to prevent certain types of headaches.

☐ Helps relieve fatigue and irritability.

☐ Promotes right Ph of bladder and vagina to maintain health.

☐ Breaks down and removes excess congestion.

☐ Makes muscles supple, helping to prevent stiffness and back-ache.

Dosage: 1 to 2 tsp. 1 to 3 x day with meals

NOURISH YOUR PITUITARY GLAND

Alfalfa Medicago sativa

I deeply appreciate this wonder of nature called alfalfa. This simple little plant sends its roots over 100 feet into the earth searching for vital minerals. Alfalfa is a luscious, abundant plant that displays a beautiful array of purple flowers. This valuable plant originally came from Persia.

I frequently use alfalfa in my practice. Two cases come to mind immediately. Both involve people whom I love. Using alfalfa in tablet form, both cases of gastro-intestinal disturbance cleared up.

Uses:

☐ Reduces acidity - high in alkaline minerals.

☐ Cleans out diverticulitis (bowel pockets) - contains a special fibre that helps to clean out toxic waste from pockets in the colon, this fibre also supports proper intestinal flora.

☐ Improves digestion - contains 8 essential enzymes.

☐ Increases quality and production of breast milk.

☐ Vitamin/Mineral supplement - contains the following nutrients: protein, calcium, phosphorus, iron, potassium, choline, sodium, silica, magnesium, 8 essential enzymes, Vitamins A, D, B6, K, U (anti-peptic ulcer) & P (rutin - bioflavonoid).

❏ Reduces water retention - is a mild diuretic.
❏ Improves assimilation by its action on the sympathetic nervous system favourably influencing nutrition. Tones up the appetite and digestion. Results in greatly improved mental and physical vigour.
❏ Helps to heal ulcers - contains significant amounts of Vit. U.
❏ Nourishes and improves pituitary function.

Caution: Alfalfa, especially in tablet form, is very drying and could aggravate Wind conditions over time. Wind need to use oil with them to prevent drying.

Dosage: Tablets or capsules - 2 to 4 with meals

NOURISH YOUR ENERGY BODY

Ginseng
(Chinese or Korean) Panax Ginseng
(Siberian) Eleutherococcus Senticsus

Ginseng is one of the most valuable herbs. Some roots sell for thousands of dollars. It is a native of Manchuria, China & other parts of east Asia. It is cultivated in China, Korea & Japan. Sadly, there are very few wild plants anymore. Please consider this when harvesting herbs and leave plenty.

Uses:

❏ Ginseng is highly prized for **its ability to rebuild you when you have been ill or run down.**
❏ It is a **tonic** par excellent. In this modern world with all its **stress** it is a valuable ally. It **nurtures your stress glands (adrenal)** enabling them to function better.
❏ Ginseng **improves performance levels** both physical & mental. Many athletes use it.
❏ It is an **adaptogen** that means it regulates a number of different body systems to keep them in **harmony.**
❏ For those of you or your patients who suffer from **fatigue** Ginseng is your herb of choice. I have seen Ginseng help many people who came to me for fatigue.
❏ It is **rejuvenating for the sexual organs** of both sexes. In the male it **increases testosterone** levels while **decreasing prostate weight.** Testosterone is a hormone that enhances male qualities. Interestingly, it **exerts oestrogen-like action** on the female reproductive system.
❏ Herbalists regard it as a **longevity** herb and studies have proven it to lengthen the life span of cells in culture.

☐ It **enhances the immune system** by **stimulating your macrophages**, the "pac-men" of your body. They filter the blood & lymph by engulfing & destroying bacteria, viruses, worn out red blood cells & other waste matter.

☐ It **protects the liver** & offers some protection against harmful **radiation**.

☐ Ginseng acts as a **hormone arouser** waking up your whole body. Its' effects last from 4 to 6 hours.

☐ It is best suited for **Wind diseases** esp. those of old age. Fire & Water can use Ginseng being careful to monitor its heating & weight increasing abilities.

☐ The Chinese consider Ginseng one of the most **yang** herbs & a **chi tonic**. Chi is our vital life force energy.

There are three ginsengs that we use. Chinese ginseng is the hottest and my choice for extreme fatigue. American ginseng is cooler and better for fire types and hotter seasons. Siberian ginseng is the best for regular use.

There are many herbs that combine well with Ginseng. They are Licorice, Orange Peel, Ginger, Elecampane & Cinnamon.

Do This!

Exercise 15 • *Increasing Your Energy with Ginseng*

Next time you are feeling a little run down, purchase some Siberian Ginseng (be certain it is authentic, preferably from Siberia. It tastes mostly bland with a slight bitter taste).

Dosage: Powder - blend 1 Tbls. in your favourite drink (preferrably not orange).
1 cup before breakfast and another in the afternoon around 3:00 P.M.
Tablet or capsule - 1 to 2 at same times
Tincture - 1-5 ml. at same times
Do this for one month. Go to bed earlier than usual if you can.

Contra indications:
Do not use if you drink a lot of coffee, you find that it elevates your blood pressure or it makes you hyper or nervous.

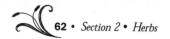

NOURISH YOUR BLOOD

Red Clover Trifolium pratense

☐ Red clover is a mild blood purifier that is suitable for general consumption and long term usage.

☐ Its taste is pleasant and it is a mildly strengthening tonic. It can be used with children, the elderly or in conditions of debility.

☐ Mineral rich helping to build strong bones, teeth and lungs.

Dosage: Strong infusion - 1 to 3 cups a day between meals

Burdock Arctium lappa

☐ Burdock cleanses the blood and lymphatics.

☐ Burdock root has nutritive properties and is eaten in Japan as a vegetable (Gobo).

☐ It is a tonic for Fire Constitutions.

☐ It is good for clearing firey emotions like anger and aggression.

Dosage: Decoction - 1 to 3 cups a day between meals

Yellow Dock Rumex crispus

☐ Yellow Dock is a good general cleanser of blood and lymph. It is good for most toxic conditions of the circulatory system.

☐ A major herb for reducing high Fire.

☐ It relieves toxic heat and clears infections.

☐ Reduces pain and inflammation.

☐ It stimulates the absorbtion of iron and helps build the blood.

Dosage: Decoction - 1 to 3 cups a day between meals

Plantain

Plantago Major - broad leaf

Plantago Lancelot - narrow leaf

This is one plant that you definitely want to get to know. It may save someone's life someday. This humble little herb's availability enhances its healing value. It grows abundantly and everywhere. I have always been able to find a fresh plantain leaf when I needed it. This is immensely important as this plant is excellent for bee stings. Plantain draws out the poison, eliminating pain and swelling, even in delicate areas like the eyes. It works very well for blood poisoning. The simplest method is to chew up a few leaves and apply directly to the afflicted area. For blood poisoning the plant should be taken internally as well.

Uses:

☐ Good for Leukaemia & Glandular disorders - purifies the blood and lymph systems.

☐ Blood poisoning, Snake bites, Stings - drawing and eliminating poisons.

☐ Relieves pain (toothache, neuralgia, etc.) - sedative for pain and the nerves.

☐ Mercurial poisoning - eliminates the poison.

☐ Vaginal disorders with discharge - clears up the infection and expels it.

☐ Bedwetting - astringent and sedative.

☐ Improves protein digestion - contains proteolytic enzymes, which breaks down proteins.

☐ Relieves stomach upset - neutralizes stomach acids and normalizes stomach secretions.

☐ Helps constipation - use seeds and husks as a laxative.

Dosage: Strong infusion - 1/2 to 1 cup 2 to 5 x day between meals
Tincture - 2 to 5 ml. 2 to 5 x day between meals

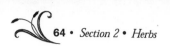

NOURISH YOUR LIVER

Dandelion Root & Leaves
Taraxacum officinale

☐ First class liver cleanser and tonic.

☐ Rich source of easily-absorbed minerals.

☐ Clears congestion of the spleen, pancreas, gall bladder, bladder and kidneys.

☐ Rich in organic sodium and of tremendous benefit to the stomach and intestines.

☐ The leaves are an excellent diuretic high in potassium which the body loses when we use diuretics.

☐ Dandelion root regulates the blood sugar and is excellent for hypoglycemia (low blood sugar).

Dosage: Decoction - 1/2 to 1 cup 2 to 5 x day with meals
            Tincture - 2 to 5 ml. 2 to 5 x day with meals

Mary's Thistle Silybum marianum

☐ Mary's Thistle is probably the best liver tonic available today. It occupies the receptor sites in the liver and cleanses the toxins therein, preventing the further uptake of poisons.

☐ It is the only remedy (botanical or otherwise) found to be effective for the deadly poisoning of *Amanita phalloides mushrooms if taken soon enough.

☐ Helpful for psoriasis.

Dosage: Tincture - 2 to 5 ml. 2 to 5 x day with meals

Oregon Grape Root Berberis aquifolium

☐ Oregon Grape Root stimulates the secretion of bile.

☐ Purifies the blood.

☐ Excellent for the treatment of skin diseases due to toxins in the blood, including psoriasis, eczema, herpes, and acne.

☐ It is a tonic for all the glands and it aids in the assimilation of nutrients.

Dosage: Decoction - 1/2 to 1 cup 2 to 5 x day with meals
            Tincture - 2 to 5 ml. 2 to 5 x day with meals

NOURISH YOUR BRAIN

Calamus Acorus calamus

☐ Calamus is a popular ayurvedic herb for the brain and nervous system.

☐ It encourages cerebral circulation, sharpens memory and enhances awareness.

☐ It is an excellent detoxifying herb especially for heavy marijuana users.

Dosage: Tincture - 2-4 ml. 2 to 5 x day after meals

Fo-Ti Polygonum multiforum

☐ Rejuvenating herb.

☐ Builds the blood and sperm.

☐ Strengthens the muscles, tendons, ligaments, and bones.

☐ It strengthens the kidneys, the liver and the nervous system.

☐ Restorative for the hair.

Dosage: Decoction - 1/2 to 1 cup 2 to 5 x day after meals
            Tincture - 2 to 5 ml. 2 to 5 x day after meals

Gota Kola Hydrocotyle asiatica

☐ Possibly the most important rejuvenating herb in Ayurvedic medicine.

☐ Revitalizes the nerves and the brain.

☐ Increases intelligence, longevity, memory and decreases senility and aging.
   Good for the prevention of Alzheimers disease.

☐ Bolsters the immune system.

☐ Nourishes the adrenal glands.

☐ Good blood purifier and helpful for chronic skin diseases.

☐ Helps the healing of wounds.

☐ Good for alcohol-induced cirrhosis of the liver.

☐ Good for all three constitutions:
                    tonic and rejuvenating for Fire.
                    inhibits Wind and calms the nerves.
                    reduces excess Water.

Dosage: Strong infusion - 1/2 to 1 cup 2 to 5 x day after meals
            Tincture - 2 to 5 ml. 2 to 5 x day after meals

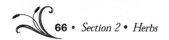

NOURISH YOUR NERVOUS SYSTEM

Oatstraw Avena sativa

☐ Oatstraw is an excellent nerve tonic, containing the essential nutrients needed for regeneration of nerve tissue.

☐ It is good for hyperactive children.

☐ Helps control bed-wetting.

☐ Restorative for burned out adults.

☐ Promotes restful sleep.

☐ Helps to prevent tension headaches.

☐ Stabilizes blood sugar and helps reduce extreme mood swings.

☐ Promotes healthy bones, teeth and lungs.

Dosage: Strong infusion - 1/2 to 1 cup 2 to 5 x day between meals
            Tincture - 2 to 5 ml. 2 to 5 x day between meals

NOURISH YOUR HEART

Hawthorn Crataegus oxyacantha

It is a healer of the heart. When I nestle in close to a Hawthorn tree and gently hug her, we both find such love and strength. When taking it as a heart remedy, I encourage you to spend time with a Hawthorn tree.

Uses:

☐ Increase intercellular Vit. C. levels by stabilizing Vit. C.

☐ Decrease capillary permeability & fragility.

☐ Collagen stabilizing action.

☐ Reduce uric acid levels.

☐ Strengthen tendons, ligaments & cartilage.

☐ Prevent free radical damage.

☐ Reduces inflammation.

☐ Exerts a mild and effective antihypertensive effect.

☐ Lessens chance of angina attacks.

☐ Reduces serum cholesterol levels.

☐ Prevents the deposition of cholesterol in the arterial walls.

☐ Reduces the size of existing atherosclerotic plaques.

☐ Improves blood supply to the heart by dilating the coronary vessels.

☐ Improves hearts metabolic processes, increasing the force of contraction and eliminates some rhythm disturbances.

☐ Promotes digestion & helps remove accumulated food masses or even tumours in the gastro-intestinal tract.

Caution: Hawthorn is safe, though people taking beta-blockers may experience mild hypertensive response from increased cardiac output.

Do This!

Exercise 16 • *Hawthorn Elixir*

Make an elixir with the berries. Buy a good bottle of brandy and empty into a wide mouth jar. Harvest or purchase enough berries to fill the jar. Shake daily for at least one month. Longer is even better. We usually do this every year. Herbalists call this a saturation tincture.

Dosage: Tincture - 2 to 5 ml. 2 to 5 x day with meals. Hawthorn can take a couple weeks to get into the tissues, so give it time.

You can also make a delicious jam. Make only enough for the year and put up in small canning jars. * Strain out all seeds.

Do This!

Exercise 17 • *Nourishing Your Heart*

Place your hand over your heart. Feel the beating of your heart. Imagine your heart sending blood full of rich oxygen and nutrition. Feel it going to every cell in your body, from the tip of your big toe to the crown of your head. Imagine all your cells bathed in this life giving fluid. Open yourself to this eternal rhythm of life affirming energy. As you breathe in imagine the blood absorbing the oxygen from your lungs and as you breathe out sense it travelling to every part of your body. When you are finished take a couple more breaths and thank your heart for it's faithful work. Ask it if it needs anything? More exercise, fresh air, iron, magnesium, Vitamin E or herbs like Hawthorn, Motherwort or Lily of the Valley?

Motherwort   Leonurus cardiaca

☐ Motherwort is a good tonic for the heart.

☐ Combined with hawthorn berries it is a very effective anti-spasmodic relieving palpitations, tachycardia and hypertension.

☐ Motherwort is a very useful herb to treat suppressed menstruation.

☐ It is excellent for calming nervous conditions. Helps with insomnia and sleep disorders.

☐ As a bitter tonic it is good for digestion.

☐ Relieves menstrual cramps.

☐ Thyroid tonic.

Dosage: Strong infusion - 1/2 to 1 cup 2 to 5 x day with meals
             Tincture - 2 to 5 ml. 2 to 5 x day with meals

Mistletoe   Viscum album

☐ Mistletoe is a first class heart remedy. It promotes elasticity in the arteries and is good for hardening of the arteries and high blood pressure.

☐ It is also good for headaches accompanied by dizziness.

Caution: Mistletoe berries are poisonous. Use only a standardised preparation and stick to the dosage listed on it.

Garlic   Allium sativum

☐ Lowers blood pressure.

☐ See Protect Yourself for more info.

☐ It is a tonic for Fire Constitutions.

☐ It is good for clearing firey emotions like anger and aggression.

Dosage: Fresh cloves - 1 to 2 cloves 2 to 5 x day with food
             Capsules - 1 to 2 capsules 2 to 5 x day with food

NOURISH YOUR MALENESS

Orange Peel Citrus resticulata

☐ Orange Peel contains precursors for the production of essential male hormones.

☐ It is a warming and decongestive herb, particularly good for the male genitals and reproductive system (common orange peels have a cooler and milder action than Mandarin orange).

Dosage: Strong infusion - 1/2 to 1 cup, 2 to 5 x day before meals
Tincture - 2 to 5 ml., 2 to 5 x day before meals

Caution: Use only organic orange peels as commercial oranges are heavily sprayed. The more aged the better.

Ginseng

See...Nourish Your Energy Body

Saw Palmetto Serenoa repens

☐ Saw Palmetto berries are one of the best herbs for the prostate gland esp. for a condition called benign prostatic hyperplasia (BPH). They act as a cleanser, decongestant, and help reduce swelling and inflammation of this important male gland.

☐ It is an excellent male tonic.

Dosage: Decoction - 1/2 to 1 cup, 2 to 5 x day before meals
Tincture - 5 ml. 2 to 5 x day before meals

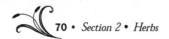

NOURISH YOUR FEMALENESS

Chaste Tree Vitex agnus castus

☐ Chaste Tree berries are rejuvenating for the female organs and reproductive system.

☐ They are a natural tonic for the **pituitary gland** regulating the whole hormonal system esp. menstrual cycle.

☐ Excellent for endometriosis and uterine fibroids.

☐ Reduces breast tenderness and lumps in the breast.

☐ Helps to regulate menstrual cycle.

☐ Helps to regulate hot flashes during menopause.

☐ Reduces estrogen and increases progesterone strengthening the vagina and bones.

☐ Reduces chronic menstrual cramps.

Dosage: Strong infusion - 1/2 to 1 cup 2 to 5 x day before meals
           Tincture - 1 ml. 2 to 5 x day before meals

False Unicorn Chamailirium luteum

☐ Used in the treatment of female sterility and impotence.

☐ We have been rewarded many times, watching this wonderful herb, help women conceive and carry to full term, when they had previously failed.

☐ Used for the treatment of menorrhea, painful menstruation, irregular menstruation and leucorrhea.

☐ Use in small amounts during the early part of pregnancy to relieve morning sickness.

Dosage: Decoction - 1/2 to 1 cup 2 to 5 x day before meals
           Tincture - 2 to 5 ml. 2 to 5 x day before meals

Caution: If a woman does **not** want to get pregnant then she should avoid false unicorn root.

Dong Quai Angelica senensis

☐ Dong Quai is a warming tonic that benefits conditions of a cold nature like menstrual cramps, irregularity, delayed flow and weakness during the menstrual period.

☐ Use to relieve hot flashes during menopause.

☐ Is a valuable blood purifier and good for the liver.

☐ It enhances circulation.

☐ Moistens the intestines to treat constipation.

☐ Dong Quai possesses highly active phytoestrogens (plant) that may act as an alternative to estrogen and are much gentler and work better within the body.

☐ Increases vaginal secretions.

Dosage: Strong infusion - 1/2 to 1 cup 2 to 5 x day before meals
          Tincture - 1 to 4 ml. 2 to 5 x day before meals

Caution: Not be used during pregnancy, excessive menstrual flow, if you have fibroids, bloating, breast tenderness, or diarrhoea. Women who are hot most of the time may find it too heating. They may benefit more from Chaste tree.

Partridge Berry (formerly Squawvine) Mitchella repens

☐ Partridge berry is useful for the treatment of water retention.

☐ Consider it very helpful for the uterus, especially to facilitate childbirth.

☐ Use it combined with crampbark, raspberry leaves and a small portion of lobelia, to prevent miscarriages.

Dosage: Strong infusion - 1/2 to 1 cup 2 to 5 x day before meals
          Tincture - 2 to 5 ml. 2 to 5 x day before meals

NOURISH YOUR BABY THROUGH YOUR BREASTS

Marshmallow Althea officinale

☐ Enriches mothers milk.

☐ Soothing to whole gastrointestinal tract.

Dosage: Decoction - 1/2 to 1 cup 2 to 5 x day before meals

Fennel   Foeniculum vulgaris

☐ Help promote milk flow for nursing mothers.

☐ Fennel seeds are one of the best herbs for digestion, strengthening "bio-fire" without aggravating Fire, stopping cramping and dispelling flatulence.

☐ Fennel seeds are excellent for digestive weakness in children or the elderly.

☐ They are calming to the nerves.

☐ They work to stop griping of purgatives.

Dosage: Strong infusion - 1/2 to 1 cup 2 to 5 x day with meals

NOURISH YOUR EYES

Eyebright   Euphrasia officinalis

☐ Stimulates the liver.

☐ Externally, the tea is an excellent eyewash, especially combined with goldenseal.

☐ Useful for inflammation of the nose and throat.

☐ Cooling to the body, reducing excess heat, which risks and can affect the eyes.

☐ Good for glaucoma internally and externally.

Dosage: Strong infusion - 1/2 to 1 cup 2 to 5 x day after meals
Tincture - 2 to 5 ml. 2 to 5 x day after meals

Bilberry   Vaccinium myrtillus

Berries:

☐ Helps prevent and treat glaucoma.

☐ Protects against cataracts and retinal degeneration.

☐ Has a stabilizing effect on collagen.

☐ Helps reduce varicose veins.

Leaves:

☐ Helps to keep blood sugars in control.

☐ Reduces uric acid which is helpful for Gout.

Dosage: Strong infusion - 1/2 to 1 cup 2 to 5 x day after meals
Tincture - 2 to 5 ml. 2 to 5 x day after meals

How to use Herbs
to make desired changes.

Herbs are amazing. People often ask me, "Do herbs work?" Herbs not only work, they heal. They live, breathe, talk, spice up our lives and beautify. One only needs to walk through an herb garden to know what I mean. Herbs are one of the most important solutions to our major health crisis. They are effective, a renewable resource, support localized economy and can be very engaging.

Herbalism is a science and an art. It is a lifetime study but can enrich your life and health from your first experience. The more that you involve yourself in the use of them the quicker you will master this wonderful craft.

By the end of this section you will be able to use herbs:

1) to stimulate	7) lower your blood sugar
2) to sedate or relax	8) encourage delivery
3) cool you down	9) stop bleeding
4) warm you up	10) ease muscle cramps
5) soothe you	11) help you urinate
6) protect you	12) clear your lungs

For dosages of herbs in this section see Appendix #1 in the back of book.

COMMON CONDITIONS

I encourage you to consider the Ayurvedic constitution of the individual and adapt the remedies as needed. A good reference is Ayurvedic Healing by David Frawley. These are simple solutions but they often are highly effective.

Acne

Herbs: Dandelion root, Burdock root, Cleavers
Time: between meals
Helpers: healing clay (internally and externally), vit A, Zinc, silica, evening primrose oil, dry skin brushing

Allergies

Herbs: Ma huang, Stinging Nettle, Goldenseal root
Time: food-with meals, sinus-after meals
Helpers: vit. C., pantothenic acid, royal jelly, raw adrenal extract

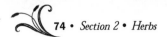

Anemia

Herbs:	Yellow dock root, Stinging Nettle, Blackberries
Time:	with meals
Helpers:	Biochemic cell salt-ferr. phos, vit. C., B 12

Arthritis

Herbs:	Devils claw, Devils club, Stinging Nettle, Alfalfa
Time:	before meals
Helpers:	alfalfa tabs, vit. C., GLA

Asthma

Herbs:	Lobelia, Ma huang, Usnea, Gum plant, Stinging Nettle, Cramp bark
Time:	after meals
Helpers:	vit. C.

Bladder problems

Herbs:	Golden seal root, Uva ursi, Buchu
Time:	before meals
Helpers:	silica

Blood pressure, high

Herbs:	Hawthorn, Garlic, Mistletoe, Motherwort
Time:	after meals
Helpers:	garlic caps

Bronchitis

Herbs:	Usnea, Gum plant, Echinacea
Time:	after meals
Helpers:	vit. C., garlic caps, eucalyptus steam, garlic oil on feet

Candida yeast infection

Herbs:	Black walnut hulls, Pau d'arco, Myrrh
Time:	before meals
Helpers:	garlic caps, caprillic acid, acidophillus

Constipation

Herbs: Licorice fern root, Cascara sagrada, Aloes, Psyllium, castor oil
Time: before meals
Helpers: aloes caps, more oil in diet, more fluids

Cough

Herbs: Lobelia, Ma huang, Usnea, Gum plant
Time: after meals
Helpers: garlic caps, slippery elm

Diabetes

Herbs: Devils club, Huckle berry, Elecampane, Dandelion root
            Golden seal root, Garlic
Time: with meals
Helpers: sucanat (organic raw sugar), vit. C., vit. A, zinc, chromium

Exhaustion

Herbs: Siberian ginseng, Ginseng, Licorice fern root
Time: with meals
Helpers: vit. C., pantothenic acid, royal jelly, raw adrenal extract

Fever

Herbs: Yarrow, Ginger, Catnip (children)
Time: after meals
Helpers: Cell salt-ferr. phos. frequently, lots of water,
            Aloe vera- if constipated

Flu

Herbs: Echinacea, Yarrow, Propolis
Time: after meals
Helpers: vit. C., vit. A, zinc

Gall bladder inflammation

Herbs: Dandelion root, Oregon grape root, Calendula, Echinacea
Time: with meals
Helpers: avoid fried foods, excess oils

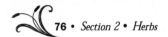

Gall bladder stones

Herbs: Dandelion root, Madder root, Tumeric
Time: with meals
Helpers: avoid fats, apple cider vinegar

Headaches

Herbs: Feverfew, Catnip, Chamomile
Time: after meals
Helpers: apple cider vinegar steam

Hypo-glycemia

Herbs: Dandelion, Licorice fern root, Siberian Ginseng root
Time: with meals
Helpers: eat small amounts of food more often, Chromium

Jaundice

Herbs: Dandelion root, Milk thistle, Goldenseal root
Time: with meals
Helpers: B complex

Kidney infection

Herbs: Goldenseal root, Propolis, Echinacea
Time: before meals
Helpers: vit. C., lots of water

Kidney stones

Herbs: Couch grass root, Madder root, Cleavers, Marshmallow root
Time: before meals
Helpers: ginger compress

Liver excess (over heated, impatient, wakes up at 2:00 am.)

Herbs: Dandelion root, Gentian root, Milk thistle
Time: with meals
Helpers: reduce fats, cut out heating foods, vent anger

Liver weakness (lethargic, grumpy, sleeps in)

Herbs: Milk thistle, Dandelion root, Maple bark
Time: with meals
Helpers: B complex

Menstruation congestion

Herbs: Pennyroyal, Dong quai, Angelica
Time: before meals
Helpers: ginger compress

Menstruation cramps

Herbs: Cramp bark, Ginger, Dong quai, Angelica
Time: before meals
Helpers: ginger compress, evening primrose oil

Menstruation delayed

Herbs: Pennyroyal, Dong quai, *caution, avoid if pregnant
Time: before meals
Helpers: ginger compress

Menstruation excess

Herbs: Yarrow, Shepherds purse
Time: before meals
Helpers: avoid heating foods

Nerve weakness

Herbs: Oatstraw, Catnip, Vervain, Skullcap
Time: after meals
Helpers: calc\mag., B vit., massage, time in nature

Prostate problems

Herbs: Saw palmetto berries
Time: before meals,
Helpers: zinc, reflexology points

Vaginal yeast infection

Herbs: Goldenseal root, Black walnut hulls, Garlic
Time: before meals
Helpers: garlic caps, avoid sugar

STIMULANTS

Coffee

I bet you are wondering what Coffee is doing in a book about herbs. Did you ever consider that it is a valuable plant? The problem is the constant spraying of Coffee with pesticides. Ask any coffee lover what a difference they experience changing from commercially chemically sprayed coffee to organically grown. The organic is much smoother, gentler and kindlier to the body.

If you are a regular coffee drinker then switch to organic. If you use a lot of cream, you may want to try soya milk instead. Some soya milks work better than others. Goat's milk is also good.

Coffee has an illustrious history from it's discovery in 600 AD by a shepherd. He noticed his young goats being particularily frisky after eating a certain berry. Until 1200 it was used as a wine or green bean decoction. Since then it has been consumed roasted. In 1600 Pope Clement VIII baptized it a christian drink. It had already been used religiously in Persia to help the faithful stay awake during their prayers. In Turkey a wife could divorce her husband if he did not supply her with enough coffee. In 1940 the coffee break was introduced in the work place. Today it is the second most traded commodity, next to oil.

Uses:

☐ Coffee is an **active brain stimulant** that many a student uses to get through finals. Some people have difficulty **waking** in the morning until they have their morning Coffee.

☐ It is useful in cases of **narcotic poisoning** keeping people from falling into a dangerous coma. In extreme cases it can be given via the rectum.

☐ Coffee **exerts a soothing action on the vascular system**, preventing a too rapid **wasting of the tissues**.

☐ It comes in handy when you have gone overboard with alcohol and need to **sober-up**.

As many of you know Coffee is **not for everyone**. It is **dosage sensitive** and quantity changes quality. **Wind** people would be better off if they **avoided Coffee**. **Fire's** need to use it in **moderation**, if they can (they crave stimulation). **Water constitution** benefits most from its use.

Do This !

Exercise 18 • *Detoxing excess Caffeine*

It is important for all regular coffee drinkers to get **lots of exercise.** Coffee is a muscle stimulant and stores in the muscles. Regular users would benefit by **fasting from Coffee 2 or 3 x a year.** A **liver cleanse** like the master cleanse is beneficial.

RELAXANTS

Catnip Nepeta cataria

Uses:

- ☐ Heat conditions (fevers) - powerful diaphoretic.
- ☐ Stomach upsets (colic, flatulence, dyspepsia) - anti-acid and sedative.
- ☐ Stress (Headaches) - calms and relaxes nervous system while neutralizing the acids created by stress.
- ☐ Teething - reduces acidity and works as a sedative.
- ☐ Bronchitis - anti-spasmodic.
- ☐ Colds - breaks up congestion, removes excess heat, aids sleep.

Do This!

Exercise 19 • *Treating a Headache with Catnip*

Next time you or a friend has a tension headache try a strong cup or two of catnip tea.

Chamomile Matricaria chamomilla

- ☐ Sedates nerve pain.
- ☐ Helps relieve bilious, digestive headaches.
- ☐ It is very balancing to the emotions.
- ☐ Strengthens the eyes.

Hops Humulus lupulus

☐ Hops are an excellent nervine and due to their bitter nature good for clearing congestion of the nervous system.

☐ They are also an excellent sedative and help to promote peaceful sleep.

☐ Good quality beer in moderation is a good hops tonic. You can use non-alcoholic beer if you prefer.

Lemon Verbena Verbena

☐ Excellent nervine, especially for nerve exhaustion due to congestion and lethargy more than hyperactivity.

☐ It is a stimulant and decongestant to the nervous system.

☐ Good for breaking a fever.

☐ As an anti-spasmotic it is good for stomach cramps and heart palpitations.

Skullcap Scutellaria lateriflora

☐ Skullcap is a good calming herb.

☐ It has specific properties for lowering high Fire. It soothes excitability and restores control.

☐ Helpful as a pain reducer.

☐ Useful for people who are going through alcohol or drug withdrawal.

☐ It is a brain tonic, good for meditation and peaceful sleep.

Valerian Valeriana officinalis

☐ Valerian is one of the best herbs for nervous disorders.

☐ It clears the nerve paths of accumulated Wind.

☐ Due to the large amounts of the earth element contained in it, it is grounding.

☐ Helps dispel vertigo, fainting and hysteria.

☐ Valerian calms muscle spasms and alleviates menstrual cramps.

☐ Promotes healthy sleep patterns.

Vervain **Verbena officinalis**

☐ Vervain is an excellent nervine. It is good for nervous conditions and headaches.

☐ Good for high stress times when you can't seem to catch up to yourself.

Do This!

Exercise 20 • *Afternoon tea break*

In the afternoon when you feel tired try a cup of one of the above herbs in place of coffee. I suggest Lemon Verbena, Vervain or Catnip.

ANTI-DEPRESSANT

St. Johnswort **Hypericum perforatum**

This beautiful little plant can be easily identified, by the hundreds of tiny holes in its leaves, when looked at from the underside. This is where it derives its name "perforatum." Hypericum refers to the rich blood-red oil locked up in its golden yellow flowers. This plant has long been a favourite of the alchemists. You can watch these yellow blossoms transform in your medicines from yellow to a deep, dark red. I personally enjoy going out each year to harvest the blossoms. I make St. Johnswort oil and tincture.

Note:

Be sure you are using the small, yellow-flowered medicinal St. John's Wort—not the large, yellow-flowered decorative garden plant.

Uses:

☐ Anti-depressant

☐ Relieves pain due to inflammation - anti-inflammatory

☐ Heals bruises, tumours, caked breasts, enlarged glands, swellings

☐ Tetanus - prevents tetanus infection

☐ Slipped disc - penetrates into the spongy material and lifts the disc up

☐ Spinal injury - relieves inflammation and is relaxing, anti-convulsive

☐ Phantom pains - used successfully in hospitals in England with amputees

☐ Haemorrhoids - anti-inflammatory and rich in bio-flavonoids

☐ Nervous disorders - sedative

☐ Bedwetting - relieves irritation, works as a sedative

☐ Herpes zoster - anti-inflammatory, vulnerary internally and externally

---

Do This!

Exercise 21 • *Making St. Johnswort Oil*

If you can harvest or purchase fresh flowers, make yourself a beautiful oil. The oil is excellent internally and externally for Wind disorders associated with the nerves. It only works with fresh flowers.

BIRTHING HERBS

Blue Cohosh   Caulophyllum thralietroides

☐ Take during the last month of pregnancy to aid in a speedy and painless delivery. My first child came into the world on the wings of blue cohosh. My wife's water bag broke but labour was being obstinate. Blue cohosh removed that stubbornness very quickly and efficiently.

☐ Because of its emmenagogue properties, it is **not to be used by pregnant women except during the last month of pregnancy**.

☐ Combine blue cohosh with black cohosh. They have complimentary properties beneficial to the nerves and a strong anti-spasmodic effect on the entire system.

STOP BLEEDING

Shepherd's Purse   Capsella bursa-pastoris

☐ Shepherd's Purse is one of the best remedies in cases of bleeding. It is very rich in vitamin K. Many midwives take it with them to home births.

☐ One cup is usually enough to stop a nose bleed. My son chews a few leaves any time he gets a nose bleed.

☐ Helps women with heavy periods.

Do This!

Exercise 22 • *Stopping a nose bleed*

Next time you or a friend have a nose bleed, try some shepherds purse. I taught my son how to identify it. When he or any of the other kids at school got a nose bleed they would pick some and eat it (with great success)! You can purchase some at an herb store.

• Record Shepherds Purse experiences

EASE MUSCLE CRAMPS

Crampbark Viburnum opulis

☐ Crampbark is of great benefit for the relief of menstrual cramps.

☐ It is also useful for the acute treatment of heart palpitations.

☐ Use whenever there is muscle tension, spasms or pain.

Black Cohosh Cimicifuga racemosa

☐ Black Cohosh is a useful anti-spasmodic for all nervous conditions, cramps and pains. I was first introduced to this herb by the late Dr. Christopher. We still use his B & B formula that has Blue cohosh, Black cohosh, Blue vervain, Skullcap & Lobelia.

☐ It is useful to relieve the pains associated with childbirth.

Black Haw Viburnum prunifolium

☐ Same as Black Cohosh but stronger.

☐ Helps prevent miscarriage when used with False Unicorn.

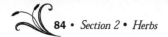

SOOTHE ITCHY SKIN

Chickweed   Stellaria media

Chickweed is found all over the world in gardens, fields, lawns, waste places and along deserted roadsides. This herb is a lush, succulent, emerald green delight both to the eyes and to the palate. I greatly appreciate chickweed for its wonderful, cooling properties. It is delicious in salads.

Uses:

☐ Trichomoniasis (vaginal infection) - reduces inflammation and helps clear up infection.

☐ Itching - soothes and heals.

☐ Liver heat (excess anger) - reduces swelling and cools.

☐ Tendonitis - loosens tightness and reduces inflammation.

☐ Constipation - gentle laxative and soothing to intestinal tract.

☐ Obesity - helps metabolize fat.

☐ Convulsions - anti-convulsive.

☐ Tumours - promotes dispersion of inflammatory deposits and their absorption into excretory paths.

☐ Hives - reduces heat and swelling.

Do This!

Exercise 23 • *Getting rid of the Itch*

Next time you or a friend are bothered by any itchy disorder, take Chickweed internally and use it externally as a wash or poultice.

SOOTHE INTESTINES

Marshmallow Root   Althea officinalis

☐ Marshmallow contains large amounts of high quality mucilage and is perhaps the best nutritive tonic herb (internally) and softening emollient (externally) in western herbalism.

☐ It is rejuvenating for Fire and Fire disorders. It alleviates inflammation.

- [ ] It soothes the lungs, kidneys, the intestines, the skin and the mucous membranes.
- [ ] It tonifies Wind.
- [ ] It is a rich source of calcium.
- [ ] It is excellent for **enriching breast milk.**
- [ ] I use it as a buffer with herbs that are somewhat irritating to soften their action e.g. Elecampane.

SOOTHE GUMS

Myrrh Commiphora myrrha

- [ ] It makes an excellent mouthwash for the gums.
- [ ] Myrrh is helpful for cases of candida yeast over growth.
- [ ] Being a resin it works deep in the tissues.
- [ ] It catalyses healing of sores and wounds, while stopping pain.
- [ ] Myrrh possesses true tonic, stimulant and rejuvenating powers.
- [ ] It is wise to use a pungent herb like Ginger to help move it through the tissues.

SOOTHE EARS

Mullein Flowers Verbascum thapsus

- [ ] It is a specific herb for mumps, earaches and glandular swellings. Mullein flowers relieve inflammation of the nerve tissue, and allay irritation.

SOOTHE SKIN

Calendula Calendula officinalis

- [ ] We have found calendula in some cases to be as effective as cortisone without the harmful side effects.
- [ ] We used it as a salve to soothe pain and irritation.
- [ ] We use it in cases of herpes, fevers, ulcers, and eruptive skin diseases.

Walnut Hulls Juglans nigra

☐ Walnut is one of the best remedies for candida.

☐ It is one of the strongest anti-fungal remedies available. It can be used externally or internally. It is great for athlete's foot.

SOOTHE EYES

Goldenseal Hydrastis canadensis

*Endangered species (use only organically grown)

☐ Goldenseal is one of the finest herbs for the eyes as an eyewash.

A native friend back east (where goldenseal grows wild) has used it regularly as an eyewash for years. Her eyes sparkle!

Do This!

Exercise 24 • *Soothing Tired Eyes*

Next time your eyes are tired and blood shot, make a tea of goldenseal. Strain well and bathe your eyes, directly or use as a compression on the eyes.

PROTECT ME Strengthen the Immune System

Echinacea Echinacea angustifoia or purpurea

Echinacea is one of my top five favourite herbs. Echinacea is the best immune stimulating herb in western herbalism. It is a natural pro-biotic (for life) compared to anti-biotic (against life). It cleanses the blood and lymph system by enhancing the action T-lymphocytes and other white blood cells. I have used Echinacea thousands of times with myself and others and have seen excellent results.

Uses:

☐ Lowered immune response - frequent colds and flus.

☐ Mononucleosis - I know of two cases that cleared up in 1/4 of the average time it takes.

☐ Bacterial and viral infection.

☐ Anti-inflammatory.

Important:

Echinacea works best if given immediately when you suspect a problem. I usually take a couple of doses when I start to feel run down as a prophylactic. It is important to take enough often enough 25 - 60 drops 4 to 5 x a day. It is important to take it for a few days after you feel better to help the body re-establish itself.

Many different experts disagree on how long you should use it. I have known people to use it for 1 1/2 years because of their extremely run down condition. A normally healthy individual usually responds right away. Children respond very favourably to it.

Remember that the sooner you ingest it the better it will work.

Propolis

Propolis is my favourite natural medicine. It is actually a by-product made by bees mostly from the sap of the popular tree. They use it to cement their hives and to embalm any sick or dead bees to protect the rest of the hive. Meat embedded with propolis is preserved since all the microbes which cause decay, are destroyed.

Uses:

☐ Propolis is an amazing ancient remedy for viral and bacterial infections.
☐ It is very useful for coughs and colds.
☐ Very effective for urinary disorders.
☐ It stimulates the immune system.
☐ Relieves the pain and helps heal stomach ulcers.

My favourite method of using propolis is dropped directly into throat or gargle in a little hot water and swallow, as many viral infections begin in the throat. I gargle as frequently as seems necessary. It soothes my throat and decreases the pain (**anaesthetic**). Propolis tincture can be made milder by adding marshmallow tincture to it.

Tincture: 15 drops in a glass of water (some resin may stick to glass, alcohol can be used to clean it - gargle if your throat is sore and then swallow).

Capsules: for stomach ulcers I fill "00" capsules with 15 drops of tincture and **use immediately**. 1 or 2 capsules before meals.

Garlic Allium sativum

Uses:

- ☐ Antibacterial
- ☐ Antifungal
- ☐ Destroys many types of worms.
- ☐ Protects against infection and promotes production of antibodies.

COOL ME DOWN

Devil's Claw Harpagophytum procumbens

- ☐ Devil's Claw has strong **anti-inflammatory** properties and is often useful in many cases of **arthritis**. We have seen some amazing results with it.

Feverfew Tanacetum parthenium

- ☐ Feverfew is a first class herb in the treatment of **migraine headaches**. It has been effective even in cases that have gone on for over 15 years.
- ☐ It is also effective during painful menstruation or premenstrual syndrome.

Gentian Gentiana lutea

- ☐ Dries up congestion.
- ☐ Sedates hyperactivity of the liver and spleen.
- ☐ It is one of the best anti-Fire herbs.

Yarrow Achillea millefolium

- ☐ Yarrow is one of my favourite cooling diaphoretics which possesses astringent and anti-spasmodic properties.
- ☐ It is good for colds, particularly those in which fever and inflammation are present.
- ☐ It stops bleeding, both internally and externally.
- ☐ Yarrow reduces excessive menstrual flow and helps ease menstrual cramps.

WARM ME UP

Ginger Zingiber officinale

Ginger is very popular & I bet most of you have already used it. Maybe when you were sick as a child your parents gave you ginger ale. Which is still a handy remedy especially if you add some Ginger tincture or strong ginger tea to it. Ginger is a great herb to know because you can find it in almost any grocery store.

The historians say that it originated in Asia. It is now cultivated in the West Indies, Jamaica & Africa. You can sprout it in your kitchen by slicing it in half & placing it in a bowl of water, so it will take root; then plant it.

Uses:

☐ Some acupuncturists maintain that it opens the gates to all the meridians.

☐ Ayurvedic healers say that it is kind to all three constitutions.

☐ It is pungent and very reliable to break up fevers & congestion.

☐ When indigestion strikes Ginger can bring fast relief.

☐ People use it with great success for all forms of nausea, including morning sickness, motion-sickness and nausea caused from chemotherapy.

☐ Pregnant women use it for nausea.

☐ When doing a sauna or sweat, Ginger will make you sweat.

☐ Ginger is penetrating and when used with other herbs will help them getting quickly & efficiently to their destination.

☐ It can be used dry or fresh. Used dry it is more stimulating and a better expectorant. Used fresh it is better for sweating & digestion.

Do This!

Exercise 25 • *Encouraging a Healthy Sweat with Ginger*

Before you have a hot bath or sauna, drink 1 or 2 cups of hot ginger tea. Notice if you sweat more.

• Record Ginger experience:

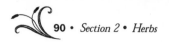

Damiana   Turnera aphrodissiaca

☐ Damiana has aphrodisiac properties that are particularly useful for women.

☐ Use when there is congestion and insufficiency due to a cold condition.

☐ It is stimulating and helps remove blocks and congestion from the female organs and reproductive system in particular.

Mugwort   Artimisia vulgaris

☐ Mugwort warms the lower abdomen and fortifies the uterus.

☐ It regulates menstruation, relieves menstrual cramping and headaches.

☐ It opens and purifies the circulatory and nervous system.

☐ It can relieve pain due to congestion.

☐ Use it in pillows to stimulate dreaming. Many people have experienced vivid dreams using mugwort dream pillows.

Pennyroyal   Mentha pulegium

☐ Pennyroyal clears the paths of the nervous and reproductive systems.

☐ It promotes menstruation and relieves spasms, dispelling obstructive Wind. It warms the uterus and relaxes the uterine muscles.

CLEANSE MY URINARY TRACT

Buchu   Agathosma betulina

☐ Buchu leaves are a strong antiseptic, diuretic and tonic for the bladder. One woman I consulted was able to avoid surgical intervention. We also use it in our kidney\bladder formula.

Cleavers   Gallium aparine

☐ Used for kidney and bladder problems, especially obstructions of the urinary organs, such as stones and gravel.

☐ It is a powerful diuretic useful in reducing weight and treating edema.

☐ It is valuable for treating skin diseases and eruptions.

☐ It's cooling properties make it a good treatment for fevers.

Juniper Juniperus communis

☐ Juniper berries are one of the best diuretics for Wind constitutions.

☐ They dispel excess Wind and improve digestion.

Pipsissewa Chimaphila umbellata

☐ Pipsissewa is useful in the treatment of urinary and genital infections.

☐ It is excellent for the treatment of skin diseases resulting from faulty elimination through the urinary tract.

OPEN UP MY BREATHING

Elecampane Inula helenium

Elecampane is a potent herb. When I offered its fresh roots to one of my students, it prompted her to write a story about "Ella," the grumpy witch. (Ella invites all the good fairies over for tea, to poison them with tea from Elecampane. The problem is, they all get healthy instead). Elecampane is one of your **best winter friends**. It is found wild in southern England, continental Europe, temperate Asia, southern Siberia and north west India. It is presently cultivated in the United States and Canada.

Uses:

☐ Elecampane is very **pungent.**

☐ When your lungs **fill with excess congestion** and you want to **break it up, move it** or **dry it out** then elecampane is your herb of choice.

☐ It can be a little harsh so it is good to combine it with **Marshmallow Root** or another **soothing herb.**

☐ Elecampane **works well with immune stimulating herbs** like Propolis, Usnea or Echinacea.

☐ It also has antiseptic and **antibacterial** properties.

Elecampane is a wonder to behold in your garden. It can grow up to 12 feet tall and its leaves are impressive.

Ma Huang (Ephedra) Ephedra sinica

☐ Ephedra is a powerful bronchial dilator and is the source of ephedrine, one of the main medicines for asthmatic attacks.

☐ It is one of the most powerful Water reducing herbs, relieving cold, mucus, cough and edema, and promoting wakefulness and activity.

☐ It relieves joint pain.

☐ Promotes peripheral circulation and cleanses the lymphatic.

Caution: Ma Huang may cause heart spasms and raise blood pressure. Avoid if pregnant or if you have high blood pressure.

LOWER MY BLOOD SUGAR

Devil's Club Oplopanax horridus

Devil's club is an important power plant of the Coast Salish of the Pacific Northwest. They use it religiously, for purification, before their bighouse dances. My native teacher, Ellen White, has taught me great respect for this herb. I have experienced desired altered states using this plant. It is not considered a hallucinogenic substance and should not be misused. I regard it as a spirit helper.

Uses:

☐ Anti-microbrial.

☐ Arthritis - anti-inflammatory and decongestant.

☐ Diabetes - hypoglycaemic (**lowers blood sugar**).

☐ Blood toxicity - strong blood purifier.

☐ Fever - strong diaphoretic.

☐ Tonic - member of the ginseng family.

☐ Dermatological aid - heals wounds, burns and infections.

☐ Used as a deodorant (powder).

☐ Digestive disturbances - digestive tonic.

☐ Colds or cough - expectorant, diaphoretic and tonic.

Caution: Devils Club lowers blood sugar so people with hypoglycemia should avoid it.

Garlic Allium sativum

☐ Lowers blood sugar.

☐ See protect me for more info.

Herbal First Aid:
The Medicine Cabinet

Bach Flower Rescue Remedy:

Shock emotional & physical. Take 4 drops immediately & give 4 drops to anyone involved. You can put it on your hands & rub onto a person in shock.

Arnica Homeopathic:

Injuries, sprains, trauma & shock 2 tablets every 2 hours. Dental work & operations same. Over-tiredness (from physical exertion) same. Sleep: take 1 tablet before bed.

Arnica Cream or Oil:

Injuries, sprains, rheumatism, sore muscles & tired feet rub into area 4 x a day. Do not apply to open wounds.

Propolis Tincture: (Natural selective antimicrobial).

Sore throat, tonsillitis, cold or flu: gargle 15 drops of propolis in water & swallow. Add to honey and swallow. Add to dry lozenges & suck. Wounds, apply directly. Stomach ulcers - 15 drops in water 3 x day. Urinary infections - same.

Ginger Capsules:

Motion sickness 1 or 2 caps before travelling. Nausea - 1 cap every 2 hours. Cramps - same. Colds, fevers & flus - same.

Cayenne Capsules:

Heart attack - prop the patient up and give 2 capsules with a glass of warm water. If necessary empty the caps into the water and administer. Haemorrhage - same as above. External bleeding - take internally and apply directly to wound. Cold feet sprinkle lightly in socks. Sprains, bruises, rheumatism and neuralgia - add to oil and rub in externally.

Goldenseal Rt. Capsules:

Anti-histamine - 1 or 2 caps every 15 min. if needed. Inflamed stomach, intestine, liver or gall bladder - 1 cap every 2 hours. Inflamed genito-urinary system, same. * **Endangered species, only use cultivated Goldenseal.**

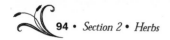

Green Clay Capsules:

Food poisoning - 1 or 2 caps every 2 hours.

Clove Oil:

Tooth ache - apply with Q tip to affected tooth. Painful sprains, rub on externally.

Peppermint Ticture:

Carminative, use 15 to 20 drops in water.

Ear Oil: (Mullein flowers, St. Johnswort and Garlic)

Ear ache - warm the oil and drop 3 to 5 drops in the ear and rub around outside the ear. It is helpful to apply gentle heat to the outside of the ear.

Lobelia Tincture: (Use with Ginger, Peppermint or Cayenne)

Asthma attack - 20 drops every 15 min. Baby convulsions - 1 or 2 drops on finger and let baby suck on it. Painful cramps and spasms - 20 to 40 drops in sweetened warm water. Earache - place a few drops of warm tincture in the ear and plug it with cotton. Difficult labour - 20 drops in warm water. Extreme muscle pain - rub tincture into affected area. Spasmodic coughing - 15 drops in warm water & sip.

Comfrey Root Tincture:

Broken bones - 15 to 20 drops 4 x day. Diarrhea - same. Internal bleeding - same. Nose bleeds - same. Do not use if you have a history of liver disorders.

Honey:

Burns - cover area completely immediately and keep covered until all pain subsides (approx. 30 to 60 min.).

Plantain Leaves (dried or fresh):

Bee stings, chew and apply to sting immediately. Leave on for as long as necessary or replace with a fresh poultice.

Ipecac Syrup:

To induce vomiting - 30 ml. (2 tbls.) followed by 4 to 5 glasses of water. Keep person walking when possible. If vomiting has not occurred in 20 min., the dose may be repeated ONCE only.

Shepherd's Purse Tincture:

Excess bleeding (internal or external) - 15 drops every 1/2 hour until bleeding stops.

CARD WITH INSTRUCTIONS:
Cross reference for immediate use.

Tools & Materials:

Scissors	Pen knife	Eye cup	Thermometer
Batteries	Tweezers	Needle	Small hot water bottle
Q-tips	Tensor- bandage	Clean cotton floss	Triangular bandage
Adhesive tape	Bandages	Butterfly bandage	Razor blade
Flashlight			

Wilderness:

Matches	Compass	Candles	Space blanket
Water purifying tabs	Flintstone	Pocket knife	Mirror
Small pot			

Do This!

Exercise 26 • *Begin Assembling Your own First Aid Kit*

Begin collecting these items and putting together a first aid kit.

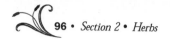

ARNICA Arnica Montana

Arnica is a beautiful, yellow flowered plant that looks like a small sunflower. Personally, I have found the medicine to be excellent in all forms of trauma or shock, especially to the muscular or skeletal systems. Many chiropractors use arnica as an oil for external use on chronic symptoms. Homeopathic arnica can be taken internally for past or present shock.

* WARNING: Arnica is toxic in large dosages and should be stored out of the reach of children.

Conditions - Healing Properties:

☐ Bruises - stimulant to the skin, promotes absorption of nutritive material and assists in carrying off the broken down tissue and promotes rapid repair.

☐ Heart strain (due to exertion and overwork) - benefits heart debility that follows severe strain, worry or excitement.

☐ Depression (deficient nervous response) - has a pronounced action upon the medulla and spinal cord.

☐ Back ache - increases circulation and nerve response.

Dosage:

Homeopathic arnica 30 X:

☐ Acute - 1 tablet every 2 hours   ☐ Chronic - 1 tablet a day

Tincture of arnica:

15 drops in 4 oz of water

☐ Acute - 1 tsp of water every hour.   ☐ Chronic - 1 tsp. of water twice daily.

External use:

☐ 1 part arnica to 5 parts water (only on unbroken skin) applied on compress, leave on over night.

* WARNING: Should the patient to whom arnica is administered appear to become nervously excited and restless or show gastric irritability, its use should be discontinued.

The Art of Practicing Herbalism

When you are beginning your study of herbs you may be eager to find people to practice on. One of the early suggestions made to me by the late Dr. Christopher was to only treat people if they have asked you for advice. I have found this to be valuable advice. If you are serious about wanting to help people with herbs, then position yourself in a place where you will have the opportunity. Get a job in an herb store or health food store.

When the situation is not an emergency, take your time to get to know the person.

Remember that the first rule is to **treat the person.** Find out what is going on with them. Make them feel comfortable. Find out which constitution they are and whether they are sama or nirama. Inquire into their lifestyle and diet to see if anything is majorly contributing to their condition. Consider what season it is and what kind of environment they spend a lot of time in. Ask if they have had any interesting dreams lately. Touch their hands to see if they are warm or cool, dry or moist. Ask them if they are usually this way.

Healing is usually taking place during the interview. Your interest, your concern and well directed questions will make the person feel better. When you offer suggestions based on your knowledge, you will usually find people receptive as it targets what they are needing. When you tell a wind person to get a massage once a week or take a hot bath at the end of the day, they usually respond positively.

Energetics: First you will need to decide whether to:

☐ tone	☐ eliminate
☐ heat	☐ cool
☐ stimulate	☐ sedate
☐ dry	☐ moisten
☐ lighten	☐ increase

Preparation: Preferably use a blend of the **main targeting herbs and helpers.** This blend could use different herbs blended as a tea, tincture or in capsules.

☐ Choose the right herb or herbal combination.
☐ Select the highest quality herbs.
☐ As a general rule, take the herbs 1 month for every year that you have had the condition you are working on.

Time: Unless otherwise specified:

☐ Take herbs for the colon, bladder or lower extremities 1/2 hour before meals.

☐ Take herbs for the stomach, liver, gall bladder, kidneys or mid-section with meals.

☐ Herbs for the lungs, bronchial, head or upper body are taken 1/2 hour after meals.

For a rejuvenating effect, take medicine in the morning, before breakfast, with soy or goat's milk.

Amount:

☐ Wind - less e.g. infusions, minimum dosage, homeopathic

☐ Fire - moderate e.g. regular dosage

☐ Water - strong e.g. maximum dosage, strong decoction

Frequency:

☐ Wind **processes food and herbs quickly,** give small amounts every 2 hrs.

☐ Fire **processes moderately fast,** give every 4 hours.

☐ Water **processes slowly,** give every 6 hours.

Carriers:

☐ Alcohol is good for transportation.

☐ Take capsules or pills with warm water.

☐ Soup is good for people who need lots of nutrition.

Important:

☐ Make it as simple and easy as you can.

☐ Play with making the herbs that become your allies a part of your life.

☐ Think of the nutritive herbs as food and include them in your diet.

☐ Imagine them saturating your cells with their wonderfully rich, nourishing energy.

☐ Learn to use them seasonally.

☐ Find out what works for you and use it. Listen to your body and your intuition.

Treat the Person, Not the Disease
Flowers Heal

In this section you will meet the incredible pioneer, Dr. Edward Bach. I personally find the essences to be extremely effective, as they get to the core of the problem. The journey through the world of feelings is a long and colourful one and the scenery keeps changing. In your work as a healer you will meet a lot of people with incredible stories to share with you and they are not all pleasant. True healing must touch the soul and to do that you sometimes need to get through some darkness. Don't beat the darkness with sticks, put in a little light. In one prison in the U.S.A. they treat their most hardened criminals by having them work in the flower gardens. After two years they notice incredible changes. I guess that is why we often bring flowers to someone who is sick.

After this section you will be able to:
  1) explain the healing philosophy of Dr. Bach.
  2) choose appropriate essences for yourself and others.

BACH FLOWER ESSENCES
Edward Bach - September 24, 1886 to November 27, 1937

Edward Bach was a determined and intense individual who possessed great powers of concentration. Bach loved the country and disliked cities. He was known for his great sense of humour, playfulness and his compassion. As a child, he dreamed of being a healer who used simple but effective remedies. He was a dreamer with intensity of purpose and two great interests: a) Healing and b) A love of nature.

By the age of 16 he had already been working for 3 years in a factory, after school each day, to help pay his way through medical school. In the factory, he gained valuable insight and understanding of human nature.

Bach found that anything that interfered with his intuitive action dissatisfied and exhausted him. While exploring both Church and medicine, he came to the conclusion that neither one fully interpreted his ideals, and so he began to look for new truths.

By the age of 20, Bach was a university medical student; there to learn what was known about healing/medicine. He spent little time with books. Instead, he spent his time studying disease by carefully watching every patient, observing the way in which each one was affected by their complaint, and seeing how these different reactions influenced the course, severity and duration of the disease. He realized that patients with a similar personality would respond to the same remedy. NOTE: the personality of the INDIVIDUAL was of even greater importance than the body, in the treatment of their malaise. Bach said of his medical degree, "It will take me five years to forget all I have been taught."

By 1913 Bach was practising medicine, but quickly became dissatisfied with orthodox treatments. He found there was little or no time to study the patients themselves; no time to think about the human side. Everyone was so concerned with the disease they ignored the personality of the individual.

Bach looked elsewhere for employment, and eventually started to work at the "Immunity School" as an Assistant Bacteriologist. Here Bach discovered that certain intestinal germs that were linked to chronic diseases, were found in everyone - whether they were healthy or 'sick'. The sick people simply possessed more of them. Bach then discovered that vaccine injected directly into the blood stream acted as a cleanser of these germs. He got great results, but disliked the injection part. He discovered that if a dose of vaccine was not repeated until the beneficial effects of the former one had worn off or become stable, he got better results with less severe reactions.

However, by 1914 Bach was in such poor health he could not enter the army. He continued working and was put in charge of 400 people. He continued conducting research from 1915 to 1919. Bach was an intense workaholic, and so in 1917 suffered a severe haemorrhage/operation. The medical experts gave him three months to live. Bach decided to make the most of the three months, so he totally submerged himself in his own work. He forgot about the illness and as a result, got stronger and stronger. After the three months had expired, he was in better health than ever!

Through his work, Bach learned that to heal any disease and meet all occasions that might arise, **you treat the patient's temperament or mood and not the disease.** The kind of illness, it's type, name and duration were of no consequence. Bach continued working on his theories around bacteria & polarity, and plants & polarity. He needed a new method of potentising (a vital point in polarity). He studied personality groups who had the same reactions mood-wise, to various diseases.

In 1919 while working at the London Homeopathic Hospital he discovered "Organon" by Hahnemann. He sat up all night and read it cover to cover and found similar discoveries. Dose repetition showed each case of illness required individual, not mass treatment. **"Treat the patient, not the disease."** "The physician's high and only mission is to restore the sick to health, to cure."

Even though Organon was going against the medical profession, Bach combined his own work with Hahnemann's. He came up with three poisons - syphilis, sycosis & psora - first two definable, third one not. He concluded that intestinal toxaemia was identical to psora. He proceeded to prepare vaccines by the homeopathic method of preparations and got excellent results. Bach found the seven bacterial groups corresponded to the seven different and definite human personalities. Through this he could diagnose the patient by personality: 7 oral vaccines & 7 Bach Nosodes. Bach was striving to bring it to such perfection of detail, so that prescribing would be possible on symptomology alone without the aid of the laboratory.

Colleagues dubbed him the second Hahnemann. Bach became so concerned with this new direction, that he dropped all other work. Bach closed down his very successful practice, destroyed everything in his laboratory and burned all his notes. He packed his suit cases and headed to the country. Bach was returning to Nature to focus only on Nature and what he found amongst the trees and plants. Remedies which were already prepared for humans by Nature herself and were only waiting to be discovered.

He rejected his earlier toxaemia work and adopted the flower essences, treating the mood and the individual person instead. **Fear of diseases was one of the greatest obstacles**, Bach found. The patients desire to get well was always the deciding factor. Bach knew moods changed day to day, even hour to hour, so in an acute disorder, he would change the remedy frequently. **Oncoming disease could even be shown by a change in mood.** This is particularly clear in children. We can usually tell when sickness is around by a change in our children's mood.

Bach's first group of remedies covered 12 states/moods - fear, terror, worry, indecision, indifference, doubt, over-concern, weakness, self-distrust, impatience, over-enthusiasm and pride. The three remedies mentioned earlier - mimulus, impatiens & clematis - made up the nucleus. Each fresh remedy needed a new bowl (the old ones were destroyed).

The remedy Cerato was from Tibet (the only plant not native to Bach's England), and was part of the second group of remedies for more persistent states of mind. Bach concluded that **an absorbing interest, a great love, a definite purpose in life, was the deciding factor of a person's happiness on earth.**

By 1934 the first 3 flower combinations for Rescue Remedy were joined They were Rock Rose, Clematis and Impatiens (Wind (Fear)/Water (indifference)/Fire (impatience)). **Bach believed all the medical training you needed was to study people and plants.** Through Bach's experiences with people, he literally began to see their spirits. He followed the thought that first came into his mind. All these years, from 1930 onward he never charged anyone for anything.

He settled in a house called "Wellsprings Sotwell". The first 19 remedies would be discovered here. Remedies 20-38 were to be discovered in a different way. For some days before discovering the remedy, Bach would suffer the disorder himself. He would then go out into the forest to find the remedy to alleviate his suffering. In this way of creative experimenting he went on to discover cherry plum, elm, pine, larch, willow, aspen, hornbeam, sweet chestnut, beech, crab apple, walnut, red chestnut, white chestnut, honeysuckle, wild rose, star of bethlehem and mustard. The white chestnut he produced using the sun method, the rest he made using the boiling method. This process of discovery took a great toll on his body, and he suffered extreme physical symptoms.

Bach became so sensitive, he could pick up on the distress of his patient coming to see him, before they arrived. Even though Bach was exhausted, it didn't stop him from seeing patients and students, and receiving correspondence from all over the world. **Bach took great joy in non medical people using his work, as he felt strongly that healing should not be in the hands of just a few people.** From this point forward he wanted to be known as an Herbalist. The medical establishment threatened to take him off of their registrar as a medical doctor (many times), and Bach's reply was to go ahead and do it. **He was far more interested in healing people than being called a medical doctor.** Even though this would have meant he could no longer visit people in their homes, it didn't really affect him, because he found people that came to see him were helped the most anyway. As it turned out, they never did remove him from their registrar.

Subsequently he trained a number of people who had been studying with him, to continue spreading his work and the 38 flower essences. He felt complete with that body of work.

Life to Bach was continuous, an unbroken stream, uninterrupted by what we call death, which merely heralded a change of condition. Bach was convinced that some work could only be done under earthly conditions, whilst spiritual conditions were necessary for certain other work. On November 27, 1937 he died in his sleep.

"I want to make it as simple as this - I am hungry, I will go and pull a lettuce from the garden for my tea; I am frightened and ill, I will take a dose of Mimulus." Edward Bach

Bach believed that the two main reasons for ill health were;
1) not following your own personal destiny.
2) harming others.

The Flower Essences:

Nourish and Open My Heart — HOLLY
☐ for love.
The less you open your heart to others, the more your heart suffers

Give Me a Sense of Direction — WILD OAT
☐ helps you to decide your aim in life.

Ease My Inner Torment — AGRIMONY
☐ inner peace, honest cheerfulness

Help Me Face the Unknown — ASPEN
☐ fearlessness, adventure

Encourage My Tolerance — BEECH
☐ acceptance, tolerating differences

Strengthen My Self Worth — CENTAURY
☐ self directed

Help Me Trust My Intuition — CERATO
☐ quiet self assurance

Support Me During This Extreme Stress — CHERRY PLUM
☐ courageous and calm

Help Me Pay Attention — CHESTNUT BUD
☐ attentive, learns from mistakes

Open Me to Service — CHICORY
☐ selfless service

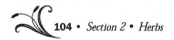

Focus My Attention — **CLEMATIS**

☐ present, curious

Help Me Feel Clean — **CRAB APPLE**

☐ broad minded, mentally disciplined

Restore My Confidence, I'm Feeling Overwhelmed — **ELM**

☐ confidence

Help Me Regain My Enthusiasm — **GENTIAN**

☐ encouragement

Restore My Faith — **GORSE**

☐ faith

Help Me to Listen — **HEATHER**

☐ selflessness

Help Me to be Present — **HONEYSUCKLE**

☐ letting go of the past

Get Me Through the Monday Morning Blues — **HORNBEAM**

☐ involvement

Find Me Some Patience, Now — **IMPATIENS**

☐ patience, acceptance

Help Me Find My Lost Self-Confidence — **LARCH**

☐ self confidence

Help Me Face My Fears — **MIMULUS**

☐ courage

End This Sudden Black Depression — **MUSTARD**

☐ joy

Help Me to Keep Going — **OAK**

☐ perseverance

Help Me With This Total Exhaustion — **OLIVE**

☐ revitalization

Rid Me of This Constant Nagging Guilt — PINE
- ☐ genuine humility

Support the Healer in Me — RED CHESTNUT
- ☐ radiate healing

Help Me Deal With This Terror — ROCK ROSE
- ☐ selfless courage

Restore My Flexible Nature — ROCK WATER
- ☐ flexible mind

Help Me Decide Between These Two — SCLERANTHUS
- ☐ stable decisiveness

Restore Order after the Trauma — STAR OF BETHLEHEM
- ☐ reordering after shock or trauma

Send Some Light into This Darkness — SWEET CHESTNUT
- ☐ acceptance of help from a higher power

Help Me Catch up to Myself — VERVAIN
- ☐ high state of flow

End This Being Right but Not Related — VINE
- ☐ sensitive leadership

Help Me Make This Change — WALNUT
- ☐ the link breaker

Help Me be More Involved — WATER VIOLET
- ☐ involvement

Help Me Still My Monkey Mind — WHITE CHESTNUT
- ☐ quiet and still mind

End This Resignation — WILD ROSE
- ☐ enthusiastic interest in life

Transform all This Resentment — WILLOW
- ☐ self responsibility

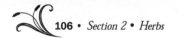

Bach Flower Essences

For further information on the remedies I recommend reading, "The Handbook of the Bach Flower Essences" by Philip Chancellor.

A couple of cases that come to mind using the essences are: a young woman came to see me for cervical cancer. The doctors wanted to do surgery and told her that she would never have children. We decided that her condition was connected to her emotions and that she would use the remedies faithfully changing them each week as needed. Her cancer cleared up and a few years later she gave birth to a beautiful girl.

Next was a school teacher who was suffering from extreme fatigue. We were using the remedy Vervain for stress, strain and over-enthusiasm. It is for people who are always one step ahead of themselves. The next time he saw me he related an incredible experience to me. He was in his garden and he felt his whole being change as he felt the two parts of himself finally merge as he experienced catching up with himself. His energy level changed and so did the direction of his life.

The last was a young woman with pre-cancerous cells in her cervix. After the session with me she decided to quit her job. About a year later while living and working in California she remembered our consultation and her condition. She went in for a pap smear and her cells were normal. I do not remember if we actually used the essences but we did use the essence of Bach's philosophy which was to follow your own path.

Some Local Pacific Northwest Essences:

The following are a number of essences that I made and experimented with over the years. For the animal, bird and mammal essences I used bone and feather instead of petals. As you may be familiar with some of these in your garden or the forest I add them as symbols for your own investigations.

Oregon
grape root: listlessness, apathy, indifference

Lavender: male\female energy balance

Rosemary: ecstacy

Calendula: steadiness of mind, maintain your own thought patterns

Plantain:	collecting negative emotions and drawing them out
Dandelion:	truth, dispelling illusions, sharing the truth
Wild rose:	cleaning up psychic energy after an abortion or miscarriage
Shepherd's purse:	psychic bleeding
Blue camas:	freeing emotions that collect in the solar plexus opening up the inner visual channel
Gold:	adaptability, relaxes excess mental energy
Arbutus:	enhancing passion, sexual or other
Cedar:	nourishment, opening up to giving and receiving
St. Johnswort:	ease the pain of separation of any kind
Dogwood:	recognising your unique beauty, inner and outer
Maple:	accepting or changing the drama in your life
Whale:	bringing subconscious blocks to the surface breaking down the isolation barrier supports group energy
Eagle:	rising above body consciousness opening up communications with the spirit world vision quest
Deer:	guardian of the spirit world easier transition to and from spirit world
Mastodon:	very yang energy helps to ground you
Robin:	rebirth, lightness and cheerfulness

Your Notes:

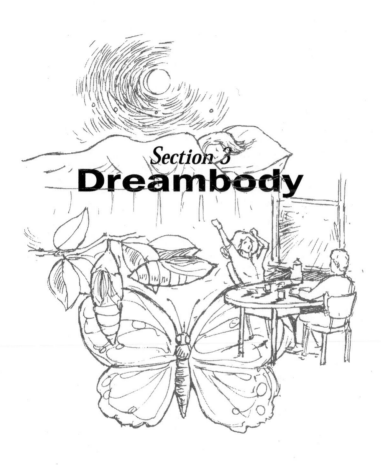

Section 3
Dreambody

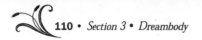
Dreambody Introduction

"Life is what happens to you while you are making other plans."
— Betty Talmadge

DREAMBODY: is a psychological system that brings together the dream world and the body. Arnold Mindell and associates from Portland, Oregon developed the concept of the dreaming body and they call it process oriented psychology.

In dreambody philosophy we think of life happening simultaneously in the material world and the dream world. The physical body has its needs as does the dreaming body. The dreaming body lets us know of its needs through our dreams, fantasies, body symptoms, spontaneous body sensations, relationship misunderstandings and synchronicities. The unseen dreaming body reveals itself in manifestations not consciously intended. Few people wake up in the morning and say, "I think I will give myself a headache today, walk into a brick wall or have a fight with my partner." These events happen to us. Our goal is to investigate these manifestations and find out what the dreaming body is trying to communicate. When we carefully examine our dreams, symptoms, accidents, synchronicities and relationship difficulties we will begin to find the same message being communicated.

Healing wisdom is weaving the material world and the dreamworld together. You will experience an increased sense of wholeness as you expand and integrate these bodies.

When working with the dreaming body we confront two realities happening simultaneously.

The first reality is our **Ordinary World**: the concrete world we perceive around us. Our plans, expectations the structures we create to live in. The way we think it is. The houses we build around us. Who we identify ourselves as. **Ordinary world** maintains our day to day. Some roles I play in my ordinary world are writer, herbalist, teacher, parent, husband and scuba instructor.

The second reality is the **Dream World**: the unexpected, the unknown, accidents, surprises and illness. Who we do not identify ourselves with. The **Dream world** is the hidden and unknown mysterious world. It may contain such roles as the poet, mystic, shaman, clown, dreamer, witch, and many others. Our spirit guardians and guides make up part of the dream world. The dream world may be contacted through our body symptoms, dreams, moods, spontaneous visions, strange sounds or voices, weird movements, etc.

Learning about and trusting the dream world more, allows the flow of life's uncontrollable events to teach and guide us. By relaxing our attachment to **ordinary world** we can open ourselves up to potential new growth. Arnold Mindell believes that one of our greatest addictions is to the idea of an ordinary world.

Most of our life in the ordinary world is caught up in linear time. We often live in a state of anxiety racing against a sense of time running out. Many of our modern illnesses are fueled by the pressures of linear time. When we enter the dream world we enter the world of non-linear, non-chronological sacred time.

Do This!
Exercise 27 • *Playing with Time*

Sit quietly. Close your eyes. Imagine that you are an eternal spirit. Let go of any need to accomplish anything. Allow yourself to just be. In this world of sacred time allow your thoughts to surface and then pass. Observe them and then let them go. See if you can locate in your body where your eternal self resides. When you find that spot allow yourself to rest there for a few minutes. Talk to this part of yourself. Does it have any advice or answers for you. I encourage you to try this every day for two weeks.

Whenever we experience pain, we have a cramped sense of time. Serious illnesses are time heavy. The domination of linear time that we have accepted in our lives is criminal. Make a habit of freeing yourself from this jailor at least once a day. More often if you are ill or suffering.

Completing this book brought me face to face with linear time. I needed to see it as a living form, in a state of becoming. It will have a form at its birth but will continue to grow and change. Your feedback will help shape its future just as our life's feedback shapes our lives.

The dreambody dreams when we are asleep and awake. Dreams and many body symptoms occur just below the threshold of our conscious mind. A dreambody process therapist or shaman helps people bring these dream messages into fuller awareness. Through this process of engaging these cutoff parts we bring them into relationship with each other. When we can integrate them, we begin to form a larger and new identity. These cutoff

parts are "dream world characters" that Arnold Mindell calls "dreamfigures."
In shamanism they are called "allies." In Jungian psychology they form
complexes or archetypes. For example, I dreamt that I was walking by a
river. As I looked into the water I saw two large sturgeon (fish). As I gazed at
them they turned into two beautiful golden seals with round faces and soft
loving eyes. Next one of them turned into a human form and crawled out of
the water and grabbed my arm. As he held my arm, he looked lovingly and
longingly into my eyes. He was a wildman all covered with long, soft, brown
hair. He wanted me to come with him into his world. In the dream I
communicated telepathically with him that I needed to move forward and
that I couldn't join him right now. In dreambody theory, I need to pick up
more of this shapeshifter power and live it in my own life. I may also grow
by reaching out lovingly to invite people into the magic of the dreaming
body. As far as shapeshifting, I still need to learn how to be more fluid with
the roles that I play.

The energy that forms dreamfigures can also reside in our bodies as
symptoms. By working with symptoms we can connect with and encourage
dreamfigures to grow and change. They are usually parts of ourselves wanting
and needing attention and development for our own and our culture's
benefit. As we get to know our dreamfigures and invite them into our
awareness through processing our dreams and body symptoms we grow and
change with them. The following exercise was developed by Arnold Mindell.

Do This!

Exercise 28 • *Processing a Body Symptom*

Feel a current body symptom that bothers you.

Describe it in detail: Is it sharp or dull? Constant or changing? Hot or cold? Localised or general?

Gently amplify the symptom according to its quality. If it is sharp then apply a sharp pressure. If it is dull then apply a dull pressure. If it is hot then make it hotter. You are taking over the function of the symptom maker. Pay careful attention to what happens as you amplify the symptom.

Does the pain move to another place? Does the pain look like something? Does the pain bring a memory or thought? Does it make you want to move?

Follow the process of change once it has begun. Where does the pain want to lead you? Get creative with your process. If you visualize something, then draw or paint it. If you move then slowly and consciously make your movements larger. If someone comes to mind then relate with that person in your imagination or in person if possible or desirable. If you have a *body feeling, then stay with the feeling. Spend some time exploring the sensation. Your body is having a dream. When you feel complete it is helpful to write down your experience or share it with a friend.

* An excellent book on body feeling is Focusing by Eugene T. Gendlin. This is a way of working with the dream world as it manifests in our body. As we observe and explore this mysterious energy, we learn more about it. Find out what it wants, act on it, change and grow.

• Record the processing of your symptom

WALKING THE PATHS OF THE SENSES

The dreambody communicates to us through **channels** or **paths**.

- ☐ Sound - auditory (inner and outer), voices, thoughts and sounds.
- ☐ Visual - inner and outer images or colours.
- ☐ Feeling - proprioceptive, body sensations.
- ☐ Movement - Kinesthesia
- ☐ Smell - oflactatory. Gustatory - taste. We combine these.
- ☐ Relationship - with yourself and other individuals.
- ☐ Community - how we are at work, in groups, in our environment etc.
- ☐ Environment - the different environments we live in.
- ☐ Spirit - unseen energies usually in the background that give us messages we can't receive from anywhere else.

These paths are either **occupied** or **unoccupied**. Julie Diamond, a dreambody process therapist from Portland, Oregon gives the following analogy: our being is like a "haunted house"; we live in and occupy certain rooms of the house. Other rooms are empty and unoccupied, and therefore become haunted by ghosts (dreamfigures). Occupied means someone is home. Unoccupied means no one is home.

Someone occupying the auditory and visual paths, may have proprioceptive (feeling) and kinesthesia (movement) paths unoccupied. They would gain the most living space by occupying the proprioceptive and kinesthesia rooms. In other words they would learn new information about themselves through feeling and movement.

Often people resist working with unoccupied paths. People who experience life through their feelings may resist thinking and space out when asked to explain what they are feeling. They may have an edge around their "intellectual" side (sound path).

"Most people think of the mind as located in the head, but the latest findings in physiology suggest that the mind doesn't really dwell in the brain but travels the whole body on caravans of hormone and enzyme, busily making sense of the compound wonders we catalogue as touch, taste, smell, hearing and vision." *A Natural History of the Senses* by Diane Ackerman.

Your senses can guide you to the paths that are most comfortable and familiar. You can use your strong sense to help you with a weaker one. Say you are strongly visual but have trouble with feelings. When feeling overwhelmed, ask yourself what the feeling looks like and describe it visually or draw it. To effectively learn the paths of the senses; you need to practice using them regularly.

Do This! Exercise 29 •
Defining Your Occupied and Unoccupied Paths

Spend the next couple of days defining which paths you are most comfortable with and use the most.

Is VISION the way you mainly perceive the world? Do you dream in colour? Do you use many visual words like "I saw" or "imagine this?" Do you describe your experiences in visual terms? You may enjoy beautiful sights and love to go to the movies. Visually your surroundings are very important to you. VISION PATH.

Maybe SOUND is your path and you love to communicate through music or the spoken word. You enjoy listening to the sounds that surround you. Noise or disturbing sounds are unbearable. SOUND PATH.

Are you good at MOVEMENT, maybe a dancer or athlete? Is it easiest for you to express your deepest thoughts non verbally by dancing or gesturing? MOVEMENT PATH.

Are you regularly filled with lots of FEELINGS or BODY SEN-SATIONS? Aware of moods, body sensations or symptoms? You really enjoy touching and being touched. You can speak with your fingers and listen with your skin. FEELING PATH.

Is SMELL one of the first things you tune into when you walk into a room? Do you love to open your spice jars and deeply inhale the fragrance? Are you attracted to perfumes and essential oils? SMELL PATH. Do you love to eat? You enjoy the lingering TASTE of the last morsel or drink you consumed. GUSTATORY PATH.

Do you prefer company to being alone? Would you prefer to work on a project with a friend? RELATIONSHIP PATH.

Maybe you work in a busy social place and you can't wait to get to work. You love wandering around your COMMUNITY talking and visiting with people. COMMUNITY PATH.

Do you sense the hidden life all round you? Do you spend time deep in thought? Do you have a rich secret fantasy life? Is your dream world active and appealing? SPIRIT PATH.

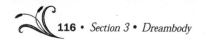

Pathways

We all walk these paths everyday of our lives. I awake from a dream and smell the morning air. There is the smell of wood smoke. It makes me feel good. Lingering in my mouth is the taste of garlic from last night's dinner. I stare up at the wooden beams above my bed. My wife and daughter lay asleep beside me, so I quietly dress and leave them sleeping.

Upstairs I turn on my full spectrum light to stimulate my pituitary. It is winter and I suffer slightly from SADS (seasonal affective disorder syndrome). Basicly it is a condition brought on by a lack of light, so the extra hour or two of artificial light makes me feel better. I take Ginseng and make my morning Coffee. The Ginseng will awaken my body over the next couple of hours and the Coffee will awaken my mind in the next half hour. My Scandinavian genes love good rich organic Coffee.

As I sip my Coffee (taste path), I feed my mind and spirit with thoughts (sound path) from some new or old favourite book. I love books. When the mood is right I sit for meditation. The form of meditation I practice is based on sitting very still and quieting the mind with the repetition of special words. Often I enjoy being still and just observing my thoughts and body feelings and allowing them to flow as they will. I enjoy meditation. I feel that my regular practice of sitting has helped me penetrate the heart of the exercises that you will find in this book. Ellen White (Shaman elder) calls meditation, preparing. She says that you never know when the door to other worlds will open so you need to be prepared.

In dreambody we practice changing paths at will. We also practice observing how our dreaming body changes paths on its own. Shamans call this stalking the dreaming body. The difference in techniques is that I am either observing the paths that my awareness is occupying without intervention or I am deliberately choosing paths to explore as I meditate.

I enjoy writing and I like to record my dreams (composite path). Dreams can be visual, auditory, feeling, movement, relationship, world or spirit. Some people actually experience taste and\or smell in their dreams. Dreams are the royal road to the dreaming body. 10% of life happens in the real world while 90% takes place in the dream world. Paying attention to our dreams can point out paths that we maybe neglecting in our waking life. If we have a strong dream about a relationship it may suggest that we need to pay more attention to the relationship path.

Speaking of the relationship path, my youngest daughter is probably awake by now and filling my morning with sunshine. She is a bright spirit. Children are life's gift to itself. Some shamans will not perform a healing ceremony without children around as they are the holders of life's future. I like the saying "For the seven generations unborn."

Next I go and turn on the computer and begin working (world path). I have developed incredible friendships (community path) over the years through my work. I hope this book will expand my connections around the globe so I can better participate in the global community.

The paths are part of our every day living. Awareness of them can be used to improve our health, reduce suffering, increase pleasure, strengthen relationships, move out of stuck states, reduce boredom and increase creativity.

Read over the following descriptions of the paths and have fun exploring them. Play is the greatest way to learn.

VISION PATH - dreams, fantasies, colours, visions.

Ordinary world visions are the primary dreams, plans and fantasies that we enter into consciously and purposefully.

Dream world visions happen to us, like fantasies that intrude upon us, disturbing and distracting us. One way to deal with dream world visions is to accept them and purposely and consciously enter them. Usually they will transform if we actively dream them onward.

eg. You have been dreaming about a friend and how much you want to connect with him. Go ahead and let yourself dream through it remembering to include the events that you imagine happening afterward. Carl Jung called this active imagination. Shamans call it awake dreaming.

Do This!
Exercise 30 • *Exploring the Vision Path*

Look around you. See what you are seeing. Look inside and see if you see anything? Think in imagery and draw your thoughts. Have your dreams presented any outstanding visuals?

• What can't you quite look at?

• What vision can't you quite imagine?

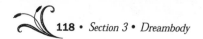

> ## *Do This!*
> ### Exercise 31 • *Visual Path Training*
> Go for a walk. Focus your visual attention on one colour. Notice where it occurs naturally and where it is used. After your walk sit still for a few minutes and sense how the colour, coloured your mood.
>
> Do the same with the five following shapes; a circle, square, triangle, cross or spiral. Do this for each colour and shape.
>
> • Record visual experiences:

SOUND PATHWAY - songs, sounds and thoughts.

Ordinary world - conscious thoughts, deliberate speech, songs.
Dream world - slips of the tongue, unwanted thoughts, inner sounds.

> ## *Do This!*
> ### Exercise 32 • *Exploring the Auditory Path*
> Sit quietly and listen to the sounds around you. Listen to your thoughts and then let them move on.
>
> • What sounds bother you?
>
> • What can't you quite hear? (Screams, laughter, yelling, noise, certain conversations).
>
> • What sound do you have trouble voicing? Try making the sound just a little.
>
> • What are your favourite thoughts? Do you have unwanted thoughts that cycle?
>
> • What is your favourite music? Your least favourite?

Do This!
Exercise 33 • *Training in the Auditory Path*
Go for a walk around your neighbourhood and focus on the different sounds. Move toward or away from sounds that catch your attention and notice which is more appealing.

• Record sound experience:

SMELL PATH

Smell is the most direct of all the senses. Smell connects with the medulla, the ancient limbic brain a mysterious, intensely emotional section in which we feel, lust and invent. This is the reptilian brain, the oldest part of our minds. Smell associates strongly with our long-term memory. There is almost no short-term memory with smells.

We have over five million olfactory cells. Some animals have as many as 200 million. We have had a long love affair with scents as some fossilized roses were dated 40 million years ago.

Ordinary world smells for many of us include the external smells of cooking, flowers or pollution etc.

Dream world smells form the hidden smells of memory and subtle perception. They include inappropriate and mysterious smells, i.e. a sweet smell in the forest without anything visible around to produce it.

Do This!
Exercise 34 • *Exploring the Olfactory Path*
Take some time out to go explore different smells in your environment. Walk around and sniff. Pick up a handful of moist earth and smell. If your sense of smell is low, take some Zinc. Wake up your nose.

• What can't you quite smell?

• Which smells turn you on or off?

• Record smell experiences:

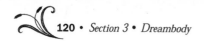

FEELING PATHWAY - touch, body sensations, moods

Ordinary world feelings: Pleasure, pain, heat, cold, fatigue.

Dream world feelings: Emotions, moods, mysterious sensations that come and go.

Our proprioceptors let us know where we are in space. They communicate about our internal organs and the movement of our limbs. They are intimately connected to movement. Touch is a powerful healer that draws us to professional hands-on healers. The lightest touch registers with our dreaming body.

I sometimes find it hard to identify and articulate exactly what I am feeling especially when I am under pressure to do so. I cultivate my emotions and value them highly. I postpone decisions if they don't feel right much to the frustration of my logical side.

In dreambody, **pain is blocked proprioception.** So before you run to the drug store when in pain I suggest you try the following exercise. Pain attempts to communicate a message from one part of us to another part. If we don't take the time to listen then the sender (pain maker) increases the pain. It does little good, long term, to kill the messenger.

Do This!

Exercise 35 • *Exploring the Proprioceptive (body feelings) Path*

Find a partner to help if possible. Locate an area where you are experiencing pain or discomfort. Have your partner place their hand gently on that area and keep it there. Your job is to stay with the feeling. If you switch paths and start to see things or enter debate, observe it then go back to your feelings. Try to stay with your feelings for at least 10 minutes. This is "cooking" a process. Whenever your attention wanders observe what was happening just before it started to wander and go back to that place. If the pain moves to another area, follow it. Take your partner's hand and move it to the new spot and go back to what you are feeling.

If something really strong comes up and you need to talk or change paths then do so.

One client of mine has difficulty getting in touch with her tears. I wrote the following piece for her.

WELL OF TEARS

I wish for you that one day you find your well of tears. The well of tears is an inexhaustible well that springs from your soul. Into this well I would lower a bucket made of the finest silver. The rope would be woven out of your broken promises and unfullfilled dreams.

Sometimes we are afraid to feel our sadness for fear that we will be engulfed by it and drown. Sadness is a well that one can safely dip into and in its waters you will find the true longings of your soul. One can easily hide behind anger or happiness but not our sadness.

Where is your well located? That is different for each person. The last time I found mine was quite by accident. A longing so deep and buried suddenly surfaced and bathed me in uncontrollable tears. My whole body cried. Yesterday, my whole body sang as I bathed in the fullfillment of that longing.

There is no chronological time in that world where the well is located. I remember those tears as if they happened yesterday although they happened years ago in Chronos world. The well you search for is a sacred well. It is found in sacred time. Sacred time is the time of the soul. My soul awakened me in the middle of the night to write these words. This is sacred time as the rest of the world sleeps. I sit alone with the fire burning writing about the well of tears.

Ellen White, my shaman teacher calls it water power. She says that I am good with water power. Maybe that is why I have touched my well of tears. Kirpal Singh, my mystic mentor, would soak his papers at work regularly from his well. So deep and constant was his contact with that well. He called it the fast road to the Beloved.

Intense longing is like an incredible magnet that draws the source of your longing irresistably to you or you to it. Like a moth to the flame, you have no choice. Reason and rationality stand no chance against the forces of your soul. May you find your well of tears and may it quicken your journey back to the beloved.

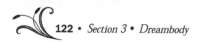

Do This!

Exercise 36 • *Training in the Propioceptive Path*

When experiencing a body sensation that you want to alter, do the following. Focus your attention fully in the sensation. After a few minutes begin to expand the feeling to the surrounding area. Establish it there and then expand it to include more area. Until your whole body is experiencing the sensation. You can do this with pleasurable sensations like an orgasm or painful ones like a headache. You can even expand it to your surrounding environment.

A change of feeling equals a change of destiny. Your body acts as an emotional filter and communicates the marks of your emotions. The reason we do most things or want most things is to get into the feeling state we hope they will produce.

• Record your feeling path experiences:

MOVEMENT PATH - how our bodies move.

Ordinary world movement: direct conscious movement, i.e. ballet, martial arts, yoga.

Dream world movement: unconscious movement: cramp, twitch, spasm, excess blinking, bumping into things.

Do This!

Exercise 37 • *Exploring the Movement Path*

Get up now and explore how your body likes to move. Put on some music if it helps.

• What movements are easy and which can't you quite make? Moving playfully, ecstatically or erotically?

Next time you are in a negative mood and you want to change it, get up and move your body purposefully and positively. A short walk is good.

• Record movement experiences:

RELATIONSHIP PATH

This path refers to our one-on-one relationships. It is a challenging path for many people and they would rather experience symptoms in their body than deal with difficulties in their relationships. Humility is vital in this path. Commitment is also needed as it takes time to work through things. When this path gets too intense it is beneficial to have outside trained help. I believe it is one of the greatest paths to growth for many people.

Ordinary world relationships - husband, wife, partner, parent, child or friend.

Dream world relationships - dreamfigures, totems or allies.

Do This!

Exercise 38 • *Relationship Path Training*

Next time that you feel in conflict with someone, suggest that you go for a walk together. Stay in relationship to each other and notice if anything changes by adding movement to the relationship path.

Next time that you have a body symptom, think about your relationships and ask yourself if this symptom has anything to do with any of your relationships? Role play, discussing what came up for you with the person in question. Notice if your symptom has changed any. If appropriate and desirable you may want to contact the person and get together to talk. The relationship path can be challenging and rewarding.

• Record relationship experiences:

COMMUNITY PATH - all my relations.

This path includes personal relationships and the world including plant, animal, and mineral relations.

Ordinary world community: The people you depend on for structure, growth, permanence and security. Architects, teachers, lawyers, parents, children, partners, bankers, doctors are all part of the rational.

Dream world community: The people who provide you with non-predictability, irrationality, inspiration, change, growth and creativity. Mystics, shamans, clowns, madmen, street people (city shadows), inventors, plant people, mineral people, etc.

Do This!

Exercise 39 • *Exploring the Community Path*

Go for a walk around your neighbourhood and observe the people who make up your community. Think about other members of your community that may not be present. Be sure to include the mineral, plant and animal communities.

• Who or what can't I relate to?

• Do you feel like a part of your community?

• What is your role in the community?

When a gypsy goes to see a doctor they take seven or eight family members with them. A strong community support system is healthy for our own immune system. In most indigenous cultures, banishment was the worst possible punishment.

• Record community experiences:

ENVIRONMENT PATH

The play of the elements around us. The sun, wind and rain. The place we find our self in.

Ordinary world environment - weather, physical atmosphere in your home.

Dream world environment - internal atmosphere, psychic atmosphere around you.

Do This!

Exercise 40 • *Exploring the Environment Path*

Think about the environment you are in, in terms of fire (temperature), water (humidity) and wind (quality of the air). Go outside and think about the weather in the same way. Do you feel good in this environment? Would you prefer a different one. Can you change your environment in any way to make it healthier for you? Add a humidifier, open the windows more or turn the heat up or down?

Do This!

Exercise 41 • *Environment Path Training*

Next time the weather bothers you pick up the energy and occupy it. For example, the cold wet rain bothers me.

So one way I might work with it is to pretend I am a big black Pacific Northwest cloud. I am laden with rain looking for somewhere to off load some. Oh, there is Don, I think I will drop some on him. I hover over Don and drop some rain on him. He goes inside so I drop more until it drips through his roof and onto him.

This is more fun than being Don, feeling sorry for himself, because it is raining again. But what about poor Don?

I then start stalking why and how the rain bothers me. We live on a boat, I start to get cabin fever, and my relationships get cramped. My wife is also bothered by the rain. Now I can go and talk with my wife, the relationship path.

So become the bothersome part of the weather and pick it up. See it, feel it, move and act like it. Next, interact as this part with yourself. Have fun bothering yourself. After you have some of the energy from the disturber, go back to being yourself and try to figure out what bothers you the most and in which path. What small changes might you make? Record environment experiences.

SPIRIT PATH

Exploration of the dream world. That part of us that strives for something larger, greater than ourselves. Our essential energy, and those energies outside ourselves.

Ordinary world spirit: What we call spirit in the world, the new age spirit, the spirit of peace, the spirit of a healthy plant, spirit of a healthy person.

Dream world spirit: scary visions, mysterious patterns, cryptic notes, devas, overpowering elemental forces or ecstatic body feelings.

Do This!

Exercise 42 • *Exploring the Path of the Spirit*

Spend some quiet time meditating on different areas of your life like your home, work place, favourite walk, parents house, etc. Can you sense a certain energy connected to each area? Is the energy light or heavy, bright or dark?

Which areas do you trance-out around? We tend to trance-out when there is an attacker around, even if it is not obvious. Trancing means you have difficulty focussing.

• Which energies are you attracted to?

• Do certain people attract you or repel you?

• Record spirit experiences:

THE CRITIC: that part of us or others, that criticizes us.

Common critics we have discovered: the **productivity critic** that criticizes us for not accomplishing enough. The **innovative critic** that speak up when we try something new. Now we suffer from the **new age critic**. It tells us we are eating an impure diet, focusing on the wrong goals, following the wrong spiritual path, or wearing the wrong crystals, etc. This can be a complex critic to deal with. It is well meaning but may come across in an overbearing, rigid manner.

We have all been criticized at some point in our lives. Since the critic often appears when we want to change and grow, we need to get to know this dreamfigure. Dreamfigures form parts of ourselves that we develop through our personal or collective histories. We can be identified or unidentified with these personalities, for example, the critic dreamfigure. Many of us suffer through the workings of this figure. We often experience being a victim of criticism.

In dreambody theory, the victim is often our **primary process**. Our **secondary process** (that which happens to us) is the criticism. When we learn to engage the critic, we can learn more about the critic process.

The **ordinary world critic** is the inner voice that tells you, " You can't do this or that. This idea is dumb; it will never work. Studying dreambody is a waste; what possible use could it be?"

The **dream world critic** manifests body symptoms like a headache or a sudden mood such as depression or anger. E.g. You are excited about a change or new development in your life and suddenly you have a headache, asthma attack or slip into a counter-productive mood.

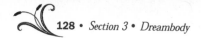

THE INNER CRITIC CARTOON

I was first introduced to this work at a workshop led by Arnold Mindell. For more information see *Stalking your Inner Critic* by Sonya Straub. Unpublished manuscript. 1990. Available from:

Process Work Centre Publications
733 N.W. Everett, Box 11
Portland. Oregon USA 97209

Do This!

Exercise 43 · • *Transforming the Inner Critic*

Create a six panel cartoon strip like the one illustrated below. Is your critic already telling you that you can't draw? Use stick figures if you need to, so you can get around the inner voice that says you have no artistic talent (the drawing critic).

In the first panel, draw yourself doing something you really want to do. In the next panel draw what might stop you. It may be a face, a voice, a big hand etc. The more you clarify the appearance of the critic the more you will learn about the critical part of your nature. In the third panel, draw the critic in complete control. In the fourth and fifth panel create some form of resolution with the critic. You may want to strike a deal. You may want to banish or kill the critic. It's up to you. Experiment and do whatever works for you now.

In the last panel illustrate your desired resolution of the situation. Perhaps you and the critic are friends. Perhaps the critic has shrunk to an insignificant size. This is a good exercise for getting in touch with and working with, the parts of us that resist change.

Do This!

Exercise 43 • *Your critic exercise*

Draw:

You doing a creative project	The critic.	The critic stopping you.
Resolution.	Resolution.	Desired outcome.

• What kind of limits are you imposing on yourself?

• Remember, argue for your limits and they are yours!

• Record your critic experience:

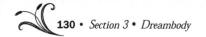

DREAMBODY GLOSSARY

DREAMBODY: is a system of healing. We use our dreams and our bodies as guides to growth. Body symptoms provide opportunities for change. We work with them as well as dreams. Dreambody brings the dream world and the body world (Ordinary world) together.

PRIMARY: refers to what we identify with. E.g. I am a man. I was born in 1946 Etc. (**Ordinary world**)

SECONDARY: happens to us. We don't identify with. Dreams, fantasies, body symptoms, accidents, synchronisities etc. (**Dream world**)

SIGNAL: is a message communicated often via dreams, fantasies, body symptoms, accidents and synchronisities

EDGE: Where we reach our limit of what we will do. Crossing over is scary. It may or may not be appropriate to go over the edge at this time. Border between Ordinary world and Dream world.

PATHS: Defined routes which we follow that are marked by many previous travellers. We will define nine paths for you.

OCCUPIED: A path is occupied when we identify with it. We are usually familiar with the scenery on these paths.

UNOCCUPIED: A path is unoccupied when we are not identified with it. On these paths we are often in new territory with new scenery.

PROCESS: A process is something that is happening all on its own. To process someone is to get involved with their process and help it along.

INTERVENTIONS: To purposely intervene in someone's process. Both amplification and forbidding are interventions.

AMPLIFICATION: is to take a body symptom, dream, fantasy or gesture and increase it by exaggerating it.

FORBIDDING: is usually a very strong way to amplify a signal. Sitting still for meditation is an example of forbidding. Stopping a movement is another.

DOUBLE SIGNAL: A double signal occurs when two messages get communicated simultaneously, usually opposing each other. E.g. Someone tells you they are not angry, but in a loud and harsh voice.

DREAMFIGURE: is a personification of a pattern of behaviours.

DREAMING UP: Dreaming up occurs when our double signals are picked up by someone or the environment and fed back to us. The person picking up the double signals is usually unaware they are doing it. They are being dreamed up.

Section 4
Shamanism

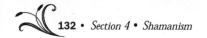

Shamanism

Shamanism is an exciting study. It can become a way of life. Where I live in the Pacific Northwest the Coast Salish natives are a shamanic culture. This includes their winter dances and pot latches. I have had the very good fortune to study with Ellen White, a coast Salish Elder.

All races have shamanic roots if we go back far enough. The labels may be different but the earth knowledge and connections are the same. Even the inner journeys all over the world have similar inner landmarks.

The training is a reconnection to Nature and to the Self. The exercises in this section are designed to connect you to the plant, element and dream worlds. Ellen White was trained from the age of seven. She is now in her 70's. I have been in training since the age of nineteen. I am now over 50. Nature is a beautiful and magical world and has many marvels to reveal when we open our spiritual eyes.

There is also a lot of power in Shamanism. We can all benefit from an addition to our personal power but be careful if you are power hungry. " What good is a power, if it stronger than you?" cautions Ellen White. When you apply yourself fully to the following exercises and practice them until they bear fruit you will be richly rewarded. Nature wants contact with us as much as we want to make contact with her.

This section will instruct and guide you to:
1) Tune into the essence of plants for guidance and healing.
2) Tune into the four elements and understand what affect they have on you.
3) Find totems for yourself from the plant, animal and element worlds.
4) Apply dreambody techniques to working with your dreams.
5) Define your bright, grey and no dreams.

PLANT DREAMWORLD:

"In long training you become one with the herbs. Connect your deepest feelings with the plant, your buddy, sister, brother or elder. How do you feel in the presence of the plant, playful, respectful, full\empty, joy\sorrow?" Ellen White.

PLANT ATTUNEMENT:

Dorothy Maclean introduced me to this incredible learning and healing tool. She was one of the three founding members of the famous community called Findhorn, in Scotland. It was her work to tune into the plant spirits to get guidance on how to grow them. She would meditate on the different plants and then write down what they communicated. Through the plants' guidance they grew incredible vegetables that attracted attention from all over the world. She taught the importance of writing down what you received. The act of writing worked to draw the plant's energy into this world.

This is the art of **awake dreaming**. First we explore dreams of the plant domain. The **practice of attuning** is vital to the **art of dreaming**. You will learn this craft quickly with practice.

This way of working with plants changed my life.

The beginning of the Herbal Healing Journey was marked by a very special event. It was the last evening of a series of evening classes I had been teaching. The students were doing their projects. The last student was my dear friend Stan Tomandl. He passed around a charcoal salve that he had made from the Devils Club plant. He asked us to place it anywhere on our body that needed healing or attention. Next he began a healing dance using two deer antlers. His dance was very entrancing and the class continued late into the evening.

Stan and I left for home in my red van. We took one look at each other and knew that we wanted to go further with the wonderful state we were experiencing. I suggested that we go to see *my* Oak tree in Beacon Hill park (a local park in Victoria, B.C., Canada) I call it my Oak tree as I had been doing intensive attunement work with it over the last few years. It was the first plant that I did an attunement with.

It was snowing as we drove into the park and parked my van. We got out and started for the tree. It was a magical night and the snow was gently falling through the giant oaks. We came over the crest of a small hill and my heart lept into my throat. There laying on the ground was my friend, the oak tree. I was stunned. Next I saw this beautiful blue glow coming from the base of the tree where it had snapped.

As I approached the tree, there was an incredible female deva bathed in blue light, hovering just above the broken stump. I gazed at her in wonderment. She smiled and spoke to me. " I called you here tonight to say goodbye. I could not leave without saying goodbye. Thank you for your love and friendship. I am now finished here and ready to move on. Goodbye."

Three weeks later the first Herbal Healing Journey was begun. I have conducted many Herbal Healing Journey Intensives since 1986 and am now expanding it to include this present work.

Plants are powerful allies that share our world with us. They are there to offer us support, guidance and healing. **Plants are the foundation of all systems of herbalism.** You can tune into plants anywhere in the world.

GUIDED PLANT MEDITATION

This exercise would work best if you had a friend guide you through it or you recorded it on a tape and played it back.

Do This!
Exercise 44 • *Guided Plant Meditation*

Find somewhere comfortable where you can sit or lay undisturbed. Warning, if done outside, the insects may disrupt your concentration. Take a few deep belly breaths to get centred and relaxed and let your body sink into the ground. When ready imagine that you are a seed. Focus your attention in the centre of the seed. Feel the seed coat surrounding you. Enjoy this deep protective internal space for a few moments (pause). Sense a slight restlessness as you feel the environment surrounding you starting to change. Slowly begin expanding allowing parts of you to reach out into the surrounding earth. Feel your tiny roots growing and penetrating. Feel them connecting and drawing in water and nutrients. Absorb this new energy and substance. Feel part of you beginning to expand upward. Feel your stock reaching up ready to penetrate the surface.

When ready allow yourself to break the surface and spread your first tender leaves. Look around at the surrounding environment. Are you in a field, on a mountain, in a garden or where? Is the sun shining or is it raining? Who are your neighbours? Feel the sunlight on your leaves and allow the magic of photosynthesis to generate new energy that you absorb. Feel the energy coming from your leaves and roots filling you. Use this energy to expand your growth upward, downward and maybe sideways. Feel your plant body growing out into the environment. Notice that buds are beginning to form. Feel them swell and unfold into flowers.

Now look at yourself. What plant are you? Look around and see\feel who is around. Maybe there are insects, birds, animals or people? Experience the interaction between you and your environment. Maybe there is an herbalist who has come to harvest some of your leaves or flowers? Sense their energy and see if you feel comfortable sharing yourself with them. Are you part of a family or are you a more solitary plant?

Sensing a change in the weather and in your self, allow your flowers to fall off and imagine your seeds beginning to ripen. Notice your leaves changing color. Begin letting your leaves fall off. Feel the seasonal change and begin to draw back into your core. It is now time to release your seeds. Does the wind come and float them away? Do they stick to the fur of a passing animal? Do the birds eat your berries and carry away your seeds? Or maybe a gardener gathers them for next year's planting? Let them go. Continue to draw deeper into your core. The weather has grown cold so withdraw to where it is warm and snuggy. Rest and relax for a bit and reflect on your experience. When complete, record your experience in words and pictures.

Do This!

Exercise 45 • *Tuning into Plant Spirits*

Choose a favourite tree. Trees are elders of the plant kingdom and usually the easiest to work with. The faculties used and developed by this exercise are your imagination and intuition. If your imagination is rusty or undisciplined, don't worry, with a little patience and practice it will reawaken. First observe your tree with all your senses. How does it smell, feel, look and taste (be certain it is not poisonous)? As you examine the tree, immerse yourself in its energy. Go slowly, gently allowing your energy field to blend with the tree's energy.

When you feel connected, you may want to present any personal concerns, emotional, mental or physical, to the tree. When I first tried this it felt awkward, strange and a little silly. That quickly changed when the tree responded. The response may be communicated in any path. It might come as a thought, sound, picture, feeling or even a movement. By amplifying the message a sound may turn into a song. A vision could be expanded into a short movie, a drawing or a painting. A feeling may open deeper layers of unexplored feelings. A movement may turn into a dance.

Since I am shy, my best experiences usually happen when I am alone or with a close friend. Sharing my experiences with a companion helps bring the experience more alive.

Once you have completed the exercise, thank the tree. Record your experience in a journal. This helps you remember, reflect and integrate your experiences.

I encourage students and clients to spend time with the herb or herbs that they are using internally, i.e. when using Hawthorn then attune with a Hawthorn tree.

• Record your plant attunement experience:

Elements:
Air, Fire, Water and Earth

When I was a young child in school studying the periodic table of elements, the teacher called the ancient people dumb because they thought there were only 4 elements. I remember very clearly how that didn't sit well with me.

They understood each element as a quality. **Earth** has the quality of solidity. **Water** the quality of flow and moistness. **Air** the quality of lightness and drying. **Fire** the quality of heating and transforming. How they interact is so revealing and fascinating. Earth without water is dry and barren. Add some water and it becomes alive and fertile. Fire from the sun can destroy our valuable herbs. Add the cooling moistening rain and the land is lush and abundant. Put fire and air together and we have droughts and forest fires.

Use this process of thinking to watch the daily changes in the weather and note how your body and mind respond to those changes. How do you feel on an exceptionally hot day? How about a very wet day? What about a windy day?

AIR

Do This!
Exercise 46 • *Exploring the Element Air*

Go to where there is a great expanse of air and possibly wind. Find a comfortable safe spot to do the exercise. Spend time exploring the air. Look at the air and the surrounding environment. Let the air touch you. Go inside and meditate on the spirit of the air. Listen to the sounds around you. Allow the spirit of the air to penetrate you. Feel it's spirit. Let it move your body. What images does it evoke? What thoughts? If it was a being what would it be? Become that being for a few minutes and experience what it means to embody the spirit of air. When ready please answer the following questions.

• What do you imagine it looks like?

• What kind of sound do you associate with it?

• What feeling or body sensation does it evoke?

Exercise continues next page

- How would you imagine it moving? You might want to try moving like it.

- How would it manifest in your personal relationships?

- What kind of work would fit this element?

- How do you imagine the energy of this element in your community?

- How would this element manifest in the spirit?

- Are you attracted or repulsed by this element?

- Do you feel you need more or less of this element in your life?

- Record your experience of air:

SPACE

Do This!

Exercise 47 • *Exploring the Element Space*

Go to where you can look out into space. Find a comfortable safe spot to do this exercise. Spend time exploring space. Look at space and the surrounding environment. Go inside and meditate on the spirit of the space. Listen to the sounds around you. Allow the spirit of space to penetrate you. Feel it's spirit. Let it move your body. What images does it evoke? What thoughts? If it was a being what would it be? Become that being for a few minutes and experience what it means to embody the spirit of space. When ready please answer the same questions used for air.

- Record your experience of space:

Do This!

Exercise 48 • *Exploring the Element Fire*

Go to where you can build a fire or be exposed to the sun. Find a comfortable safe spot to do the exercise. Spend time exploring the fire. Look at the fire and the surrounding environment. Gently feel the fire with your skin. Go inside and meditate on the spirit of the fire. Listen to the sound of the fire. Allow the spirit of the fire to penetrate you. Feel its spirit. Let it move your body. What images does it evoke? What thoughts? If it was a being what would it be? Become that being for a few minutes and experience what it means to embody the spirit of fire. When ready please answer the following questions.

• What do you imagine it looks like?

• What kind of sound do you associate with it?

• What feeling or body sensation does it evoke?

• How would you imagine it moving? You might want to try moving like it.

• How would it manifest in your personal relationships?

• What kind of work would fit this element?

• How do you imagine the energy of this element in your community?

• How would this element manifest in the spirit?

• Are you attracted or repulsed by this element?

• Do you feel you need more or less of this element in your life?

• Record your experience of fire:

WATER

Do This!

Exercise 49 • *Exploring the Element Water*

Go to a body of water near your home, a river, lake or ocean. Find a comfortable safe spot to do the exercise. Spend time exploring the water. Look at the water and the surrounding environment. Touch the water. Go inside and meditate on the spirit of the water. Listen to the sounds around you. Allow the spirit of the water to penetrate you. Feel its spirit. Let it move your body. What images does it evoke? What thoughts? If it was a being what would it be? Become that being for a few minutes and experience what it means to embody the spirit of water. When ready please answer the following questions.

• What do you imagine it looks like?

• What kind of sound do you associate with it?

• What feeling or body sensation does it evoke?

• How would you imagine it moving? You might want to try moving like it.

• How would it manifest in your personal relationships?

• What kind of work would fit this element?

• How do you imagine the energy of this element in your community?

• How would this element manifest in the spirit?

• Are you attracted or repulsed by this element?

• Do you feel you need more or less of this element in your life?

• Record your experiences of water:

Do This!

Exercise 50 • *Exploring the Element Earth*

Go to where you can lay on the ground. Find a comfortable safe spot to do this exercise. Spend time exploring the earth. Look at the earth and the surrounding environment. Touch the earth and smell it. Go inside and meditate on the spirit of the earth. Listen to the sounds around you. Allow the spirit of the earth to penetrate you. Feel its spirit. Let it move your body. What images does it evoke? What thoughts? If it was a being what would it be? Become that being for a few minutes and experience what it means to embody the spirit of earth. When ready please answer the following questions.

• What do you imagine it looks like?

• What kind of sound do you associate with it?

• What feeling or body sensation does it evoke?

• How would you imagine it moving? You might want to try moving like it.

• How would it manifest in your personal relationships?

• What kind of work would fit this element?

• How do you imagine the energy of this element in your community?

• How would this element manifest in the spirit?

• Are you attracted or repulsed by this element?

• Do you feel you need more or less of this element in your life?

• Record your experiences of earth:

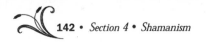

Totems

Totemism is a highly developed system in many indigenous cultures. Animals are here to support, guide and sometimes challenge us. We can encounter them in the ordinary world, e.g. My partner Sandy took the garbage out one day and there was a deer in our front yard. We lived in the heart of the city, miles away from any deer habitat.

At other times we experience them in the dream world. A common way is meeting an animal in our dreams.

We learn new ways to live in the world from our animal brothers and sisters. I have been studying and working with the power of the Canada Goose. One winter I was able to go south and was empowered by the experience. When you invoke the power of an animal you tap into its strengths and patterns. It is good to enter this relationship with reverence and humility. It is best if you can actually observe your totem animal. Some totem animals stay with us for a long time, others can be called upon for certain situations and then released.

Some animals are shape shifters meaning they can change form at will. In the dreamworld I met a whale and a bull who both changed into human form to communicate with me and then went back into their original form.

Do This!

Exercise 51 • *Finding a Totem*

Think about your dreams. Have you dreamed about any animals lately? Strong dream? What animal are you attracted to? Why? If you were an animal which one would you be? Why?

If you have not dreamed of an animal lately then ask your dreams to show you your totem animal. Be patient, sometimes the dreamworld waits until you are ready.

Do This!

Exercise 52 • *Working with Your Totem*

Find a body feeling or sensation. Amplify the sensation by focusing on it and adding pressure or slight movement if helpful. Draw a picture of an animal that matches the feeling. Does it make a sound? Make that sound. What kind of movement does it make? Make the movements. Increase the movements gradually. As you move like it, become the animal and sense its power.

We practice entering paths at will and discovering our totems. By exploring different paths, we get new information about our bodies, psyches and expand our identity.

Do This!

Exercise 53 • *Visual Representation of Your Totems*

Draw a picture with a representation from the plant, animal and elemental world. Today, mine might have an Otter, a Coffee plant and the Sun in it. If drawing is too difficult then make a collage.

• Draw a picture or do a collage:

• Record your totem experiences:

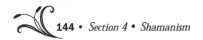

DREAMS

Before going to a large herb conference to speak about our school, the Herbal Healing Journey, I dreamed that I spoke last. There were only a few people left in the audience.

When I went to the conference I requested to speak first or second. They agreed and I spoke to a full room. When the last person on the panel spoke there were only a few people left.

Do This!

Exercise 54 • *Working with Dreams Using All the Paths* Write your dreams down in a dream journal, the voice path. Discuss your dreams with a close friend, someone who cares about you and your dreams. Ask them what stands out for them in the dream or in the telling of the dream, relationship path. Draw your dreams, vision path. Dance or move your dreams, the movement path. What feelings are invoked, the feeling path. As you work with your dream and feel you know what it is telling you, then act on it out in the world, the community path.

LIGHT DREAM\DARK DREAM\NO DREAM

☐ A **light dream** is something that touches and ignites the core of your being causing your cells to sing.

☐ A **dark dream** is a frog at the bottom of a dark well croaking a mournful song that causes your cells to collapse in resignation.

☐ A **no dream** is Buddha at a night club dancing and drinking without attachment.

Do This!

Exercise 55 • *Working with Your Life Dreams*

Imagine the most optimistic future you can for your self. Stay with this vision as long as you can. This is your light dream. Write down your light dream.

Imagine the future as an impossible. This is a dark dream. Drop attachment to either dream. This is a no dream.

• Record your experience:

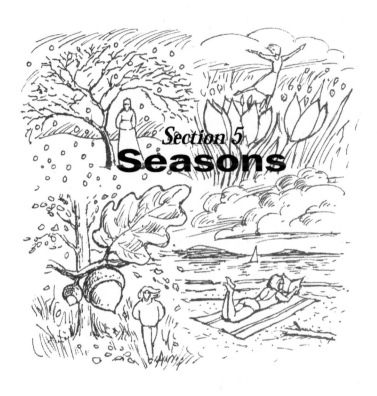

Section 5
Seasons

The Seasons

*The interaction of the five elements brings harmony and
everything is in order. At the end of one year the sun has
completed its course and everything starts anew with the first
season, which is the beginning of spring. This system is
comparable to a ring which has neither beginning or end.*
—Nei Ching

SEASONAL PERSPECTIVE

My goal is to provide you with a seasonal format for studying and living
that will be easily adopted into your life. Each year you can practice the parts
of the Herbal Healing Journey that appeal to you and deepen your
understanding, while improving your overall well-being.

In our modern world of constant change and instability I hope that you
will find some security and comfort in the timeless cycle of the seasons.

After this section you will be able to :
  1) know which organs and meridians are active during each season.
  2) use different tools to explore, strengthen and heal the different organs.
  3) choose a diet appropriate to each season.*
  4) better sense your relationship and adaptability to the seasons.
  5) be more observant and aware of the changes happening.

* Staying Healthy with the Seasons by Elson M. Haas, M.D.

Spring

Spring is nature's season of birth, restoring everything to life. Our winter dreams surface and begin to bloom. Spring is new beginnings. It is time to clear out the past. Clean up your environment and your self. Dig into the closets, basements and attics. The best time of the year for a body cleanse.

Do This!
Exercise 56 • *Exploring the First Day of Spring*

Plan to spend part of your day on or close to March 21st outside. Walk around and observe your environment. Check out the plants, animals, birds and people. Sense the play of the elements at this time.

- How do you experience the increase of fire in your environment and body?

- How is the lengthening of the day affecting your mood and sleep patterns?

- Do you feel more or less energetic?

- What kind of thoughts or fantasies fill your mind during these early days of Spring?

SPRING ACTIVITIES
Cleansing

What is cleansing and why do we cleanse?

We cleanse to clear out congestion from our bodies. We cleanse to prevent a build up of congestion that is the breeding ground for many pathogens. Cleansing releases and flushes out physical, mental and emotional toxins helping to restore our natural energy level.

Cleansing can be used during a **right of passage**. It produces a **separation** from ordinary experience. It can provide a **threshold experience**, where a peak will be reached and after that a new **integration** found.

When ill, slow or stop your regular interactions with the world. Disease processes frequently contain information for us. Our modern culture wants us to ignore or silence this information with drugs or surgery. Disease causes disruption to our everyday life. This disruption affords us the opportunity to change and reorder to a new structure. Sometimes heroic measures like fasting may be needed to move us past the point of dissipation to integration.

Cleansing helps us deal with addictions in a positive and gentle way. The addictive dreamfigure can be coaxed into the cleanse. Whatever the addiction, the body will benefit from a break from it. We can renegotiate after the cleanse to see if it is time to give up the addiction permanently.

As the seasons gently flow into one another cleansing is easiest and most beneficial at the transition. Many indigenous cultures cleanse in the Spring. Nature brings the heavy accumulated toxins (Congestion) to the surface. As we delight in the ritual of Spring cleaning, we can delight in a body cleanse. I find that a fast at this time helps to balance my Fire constitution. I look forward to fasting each Spring. I think about ways that I can improve the cleanse and make it more enjoyable.

THREE SPRING CLEANSES
Clay

"Our Earth, the oldest healer, mother of all plants, is alive and providing health to the people." Micheal Abehsera

Clay can be marvellously effective as a healing agent. It restores organic functions to deficient organs by acting as a **catalyst**, helping them to fix needed elements. It can be used externally as a poultice, or internally. **The clay should be obtained from a herbalist or any other source that can guarantee the clay has not been treated, baked or added to in any way.** Green clay is the most common, but red, yellow, grey, and white clay are available and may be desired. Clay has the magical property of being part of the earth and when in contact with your body is connecting your process to the planet. Clay is a strong healer. Clay goes to where it is needed. It adapts itself to the needs of the body. Clay is alive and helps generate and maintain life.

Clay:

- [ ] carries a negative charge (-) giving it an electrical attraction for positively charged toxins (+).
- [ ] has a large (-) charged surface for attracting lots of (+) charged toxins.
- [ ] has a strong absorbent action. It has the power to attract, absorb and stimulate the elimination of toxic and non-useful elements.
- [ ] eliminates harmful bacteria.
- [ ] removes gas.
- [ ] retains and transmits a considerable amount of energy from the large and powerful magnetic entity of the Earth.
- [ ] oxidizes and fixes free oxygen.
- [ ] neutralizes poisons.
- [ ] is a powerful **antidote** for **food poisoning**. For emergency treatment, take one teaspoon in water every hour for six hours.
- [ ] neutralizes nitrogenous wastes and eliminates acids creating a favourable pH of the blood

Using Clay Internally:

For internal use I recommend green clay. One teaspoon a day in a glass of water is an adult dosage. Green clay is a fine greasy clay that is not gritty in the teeth. Important, clay **should always be in contact with stable materials such as enamel, earthenware, porcelain, wood, or glass, never metal (aluminium, copper, stainless steel, iron) or plastic.** Therefore use a wooden spoon or your fingers to put the clay in the glass. At first you may only want to consume the clay water leaving the sediment in the glass. After a week the **Fire** and **Wind** constitutions may take the sediment as well. The person with a Water constitution has enough water and earth in their constitution already and will not benefit from the sediment. If you are in confusion about your constitution, see the Constitution Questionnaire at the beginning of AYURVEDA.

It is best to take the clay before going to bed at night or in the morning **one hour** before eating. Clay can be taken 15 or 20 minutes before eating if necessary or **two hours** after eating. Clay tends to cause constipation if taken before breakfast. To remedy this, take small portions of the clay water during the day. Or switch to taking clay before bedtime. Take a laxative tea if necessary. To counteract the binding effect of clay drink lots of liquid between meals. I recommend four glasses of lemon water each day of taking clay internally. Adding maple syrup to your lemon water will temper it's sour taste. An excess of sour may upset Fire constitution.

Continue taking clay internally daily for three weeks. Then every week alternate until there is no appetite for the clay. You are listening to your body.

The External Clay Pack:

This is a very powerful way to treat the body. As such it should be preceded by laxative teas, simplified diet and taking clay orally to reduce the build up of toxins.

The same rules apply when mixing clay up for external use. Use porcelain or wooden bowls and implements, never plastic or metal. Remember that clay is very sensitive to what it contacts.

Clay can be put on; the large or small intestines, kidneys, spleen or liver. It can be applied to sprains bruises bumps and fractures. Mix the clay with water or oil and keep the mixture damp. If the area in question needs heat then the clay can be heated. Warm clay in a ceramic bowl, preferably in the sun. Clay exposed to the sun is more active. Clay can be warmed on a radiator or a stove if it's container is sitting in a larger bowl of water. The temperature of the poultice is determined by the organ to be treated. If the organ is inflamed, a cold poultice is in order and the normal temperature of the clay will be sufficient. For example, the liver will often respond well to a cold poultice. In other areas; notably the lower abdomen, a warm poultice is better tolerated.

Do This!
Exercise 57 • *Using a clay pack*

- Measure the area to be poulticed and prepare for that area.

- Figure out whether cooling or heating is necessary.

- Use a towel or cabbage leaf for the poultice (a cabbage leaf holds water longer).

- A poultice can be used for any part of the body.

- Some organs such as the liver should be poulticed at night as it is most active from 11:00 pm. to 3:00 am.

- The thickness of the clay pack applied may vary according to the amount of time it will be left on. The longer left on, the thicker the poultice.

- Wait at least two hours after eating before putting on a cold poultice. A hot one can be put on after one hour.

- Apply only one poultice daily.

The effects of this treatment vary. There may be a flaring up of the problem due to the cleansing action of the clay. This is a temporary but beneficial effect. You need to use your intuition and vary the treatment according to the body'feedback. There is a link between clay and the dream world. There can be an emotional reaction from the poultice.

- Record clay experiences:

THE LEMON CLEANSE

Lemon water is important for its natural hydrochloric acid that the liver converts into some 6 billion different enzymes, easier than any other substance. The lemon and maple syrup mixture contains 49% **potassium**. It strengthens and energizes the heart. It also stimulates and builds up the kidneys and adrenal glands.

Its **oxygen** builds vitality. Its **carbon** acts as a motor stimulant. **Hydrogen** activates the sensory nerves and calcium strengthens the lungs. **Phosphorous** knits the bones and stimulates and nourishes the brain. **Sodium** encourages tissue regeneration and **magnesium** alkalizes the blood. **Iron** builds red corpuscles and **chlorine** cleans blood plasma. **Silica** aids the thyroid.

Do This!

Exercise 58 • *The Lemon Cleanse*

Eat only fruits and vegetables for three to ten days depending on your constitution, time, present health and inclination. During this time drink 3 to 6 glasses of the lemon cleanse. The basic recipe for the lemon cleanse is:

> 2 tablespoons of lemon juice (organic lemons are recommended)
> 1-2 tablespoons of maple syrup (organic, grade "C")
> 1 tablespoon of olive oil
> 1/10 a teaspoon of cayenne or ginger
> (ginger may be less disturbing to the Fire Constitution)

For a more thorough cleanse you may want to do the following. Each morning of the fast: mix two teaspoons of salt (preferably organic sea salt) with a quart of warm water. Drink this mixture before taking your first glass of lemon water. This will gradually wash out impurities in your system. Wait for the purge, it will come. If this process becomes very painful ease up on your consumption of salt water. During my last fast, I only did the salt water purge on about the 5th day. It worked!

Fasting Times for the Constitutions:

Fasting creates harmony between our inner and outer lives. We need mental and physical clarity to make clear decisions. Our creative self gets the greatest impetus during Spring. It is important not to disturb your constitution.

Most Beneficial Amount of Fasting Time:

The **Wind** person would benefit from no more than **four** days.
The **Fire** person may fast **five to seven** days.
The **Water** person may fast **seven to ten** days or longer.

Re-introducing Food:

Begin with soft, well digested food such as a rice pudding or break your fast with clear soup. Take it slow and give your body time to get used to digesting full meals again.

MENTAL FASTING

Do This!
Exercise 59 • *Mental Fast*

Reduce intake of new information. Process what you already have. Do some free flow writing. Sort, sift and discard irrelevant information.

• Record both fasting experiences:

SKIN BRUSHING

Feeling takes place in the second layer of skin. The top layer is mainly composed of dead skin cells. I have heard that safe crackers file down their finger tips to make them more sensitive. You will enjoy the new sense of pleasure that you experience after skin brushing regularly.

The skin is the largest organ in the body and occupies the largest sensory portion of the brain. It weighs from six to ten pounds. It is the major eliminative organ that removes up to one-third of the impurities of the body! When the skin is clogged it puts strain on the liver and kidneys.

When skin brushing use a skin brush, loofah or ayate cloth (a rough cloth). Brush the body with firm motions from the feet up to the head. Avoid the sensitive parts of the body, the face, inner thighs and breasts. Brush for a short time (five to ten minutes), then rinse the dead skin particles off in the shower.

Skin brushing makes the skin alive. Brings blood to the surface and activates the nerve endings all over the body. After a session of brushing and showering try putting aloe vera juice on the skin. It contributes to the acid mantle of the skin. If you have very dry skin then apply a natural oil. Coconut oil is good as it washes out of clothing afterward.

Skin brush daily and remember to wear natural fibres for clothing such as cotton, wool and silk. Synthetic clothing is hard on your skin because it doesn't allow it to breathe. Now that your skin is alive experience more with the wonderful sensation of touch. Let the sun and the wind caress your skin. Spend more time naked if you are comfortable with that. Be sure to touch your loved ones often to assure them of your love. Touch is a stronger communicator than words.

Do This!

Exercise 60 • *Skin Brushing with a Twist*

Brush one half of your body (left or right) from your feet to your head but not your head. Set your brush down for a couple of minutes and sense how you feel. Then brush the other half .

• Record your skin brushing experience:

This activates the different hemispheres of the brain. Brushing the left side activates the right brain. Brushing the right side activates the left brain.

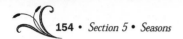

SKIN PROBLEMS

(Ayurveda Differentiation)

Fire

Symptoms:
- ☐ redness, swelling, fever, infection and irritability.
- ☐ aggravated by heat or exposure to sun application of oils.

Treatment:
- ☐ avoid possible allergens, nightshade family, tomatoes, peaches, strawberries and sour dairy products.
- ☐ avoid heat and sun.
- ☐ apply coconut oil, aloe gel or ghee (clarified butter).
- ☐ use blood purifiers like Burdock, Plantain or Red Clover.
- ☐ cleanse the liver.

Wind

Symptoms:
- ☐ dry, scaly, itchy skin accompanied with distention and constipation.
- ☐ aggravated by wind and dryness.

Treatment:
- ☐ take extra oil in the diet. We have found evening primrose oil capsules taken internally and applied externally to be excellent. Flax seed oil is also excellent. Ayurveda recommends sesame oil.
- ☐ use laxatives like castor oil or use an oil enema (see Fall section).
- ☐ lots of hugs and touching.

Water

Symptoms:
- ☐ oozing or weeping sores with congestion, edema and itch.
- ☐ aggravated by dampness and coldness, application or consumption of oils.

Treatment:
- ☐ avoid heavy, greasy and oily food particularly cheese and yoghurt.
- ☐ avoid oil externally and internally.
- ☐ dry brush massage would be excellent.

SPRING HERBS

During Spring we lean towards cleansing herbs. Number one is fresh nettle greens. Next I focus on the young Horsetails for a great Spring tea (DO NOT EAT). My other favourites are Dandelion root and leaves, Milk Thistle and Gentian. Usually I focus on a clay treatment followed by a fast.

SKIN DREAMBODY

Skin defines our boundary of who we are. Our remarkable armour, container and major sensory organ.

Do This!

Exercise 61 • *Defining Our Personal Boundaries*

Find a friend. Stand facing each other. Now one of you take three paces back. The person who took the backward paces is going to be the active person. The person who is standing still is going to initiate contact. Preferably close your eyes and sense the other person. When you feel comfortable then signal them with a nod of your head to take one step towards you.

Once they have taken that step, sense their presence again. When ready give them a nod and they advance one more step. You can stop at any point in this exercise. When comfortable give them another nod. Now they will be standing right in front of you. If appropriate, give them one more nod and let them give you a hug.

When ready change positions and repeat the above. This can be a strong exercise for anyone who has experienced abuse issues. Use discretion and go very slowly.

I have found this exercise extremely helpful for participation in groups. It empowers my body to help me decide whom I feel comfortable with and whom I do not. Generally it has made me more comfortable with others.

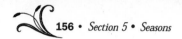

SPRING BODY SYSTEMS

Liver: Yin

- ☐ may hold suppressed anger that can be injurous.
- ☐ craves sour taste.
- ☐ can regenerate itself.
- ☐ is a master laboratory which stores and distributes nourishment for the entire body.
- ☐ is involved in the formation of blood.
- ☐ filters toxins (unusable materials).
- ☐ makes bile (emulsifies fats).

> bile: greenish yellow liquid that contains water, bile salts, bilirubin, cholesterol, fatty acids, lecithin and some inorganic salts. The inability to clear bilirubin turns the eyes and skin a greenish yellow.

- ☐ helps to keep the blood sugar regulated by changing fats (lipids) and proteins (amino acids) into glucose and back again for storage.
- ☐ forms many gamma globulins and plasma proteins that help the body's defence systems.
- ☐ manufactures enzymes.
- ☐ helps with blood clotting (pro-thrombin).
- ☐ prevents abnormal clotting (heparin and antithrombin).
- ☐ can form Vitamin A and store it with Vitamin D and B complex.
- ☐ stores copper, zinc and iron.
- ☐ turns nitrogen waste into urea (for the kidneys).
- ☐ deactivates hormones - thyroid and sex hormones.

Gall Bladder: Yang

- ☐ stores and secretes bile.
- ☐ concentrates the bile.

Symptoms of Possible Malfunction of Liver\Gall Bladder:

- ☐ gas and cramping in the upper right abdomen.
- ☐ referred pains to back and between the shoulder blades.
- ☐ pain in the hips and thighs.
- ☐ headaches.
- ☐ trouble with the eyes.

LIVER DREAMBODY

Do This!

Exercise 62 • *Exploring What Dreams May Be Connected to Your Liver*

Place your hand on your liver just below your lower right ribs. Press gently on it and breath slowly. Play with different pressures and pay attention to anything that comes up. You may just want to maintain a comfortable pressure and focus more on what comes up in the different paths.

• Record Your Experience:

SPRING ELEMENTS
Wood Element

In Chinese medicine, the wood element rules the spine, limbs and joints.

An imbalance in the wood element may cause:
☐ spinal problems.
☐ poor flexibility.
☐ weak rooted, inability to settle down.

An attraction or repulsion to the colour green may show a wood imbalance. Having wood in balance enables us to have mental clarity with an ability to focus, plan and make decisions.

Weakness in the wood element is indicated by:
☐ poor judgement.
☐ bad planning.
☐ disorganization.
☐ inability to make decisions.

When the wood element is over-developed:
☐ there is excess mentality.
☐ may try to organize everything and everyone.
☐ have difficulty relaxing.
☐ prone to headaches, neck and back tension.
☐ people with a healthy wood element are early risers.
☐ unhealthy wood makes for a sluggish, slow morning riser.

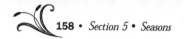

SPRING PLANT WALK

Do This!

Exercise 63 • *Observing the Plants During Spring*

Go out and observe the local plants in spring. Notice how they respond to the energy of Spring.

SPRING DIET

My all time favourite Spring food is stinging nettles. My body cells seem to drink in the power of this herb. It is a strong food and often initiates a cleansing response with me. I start to add lemon drinks to my diet in preparation for my Spring fast. As the days warm up I eat less starches and proteins.

A powerful healing spring food is Ghee (clarified butter) made from fresh cream taken from free range (drug free) cows eating the new spring grass. We have such a powerful dairy association that it is impossible to buy directly from the farm here. If anyone has access to this type of butter (I will make it into ghee) please write me and we can negotiate. Ghee keeps for a long time so you can make enough in the spring for the year.

This is the best time to grow wheat, barley or oat grass. Harvest it when 3 or 4 inches and blend into drinks. Go easy at first as this is another powerful food. Sprouts are healthiest at this time of year.

Lots of the herbs will be sprouting up and many of them are tender and succulent at this time. This morning April 7th I was munching on young willow leaves. They were tender and lacked the bitter taste of salicin that they develop later on. Those of you with gardens can enjoy the early volunteers.

Summer

My favourite time of the year. The sun is hot and the days long and bright. People strip off their heavy clothing and put on their shorts and bathing suits. The lakes and the ocean beckon me to come and play. People come out of their houses and there is more social time.

The sun feels warm and healing on the skin. It is easier to spend time outside.

Do This!

Exercise 64 • *Exploring the First Day of Summer*

Plan to spend part of your day on or close to June 21st outside. Walk around and observe your environment. Check out the plants, animals, birds and people. Sense the play of the elements at this time.

- How do you experience the increase of fire in your environment and body?

- How is the lengthening of the day affecting your mood and sleep patterns?

- Do you feel more or less energetic?

- What kind of thoughts or fantasies fill your mind during these early days of summer?

SUMMER BODY SYSTEMS

Heart: Yin

☐ pumps the blood, carrying warmth, oxygen and nutrients through our body.

☐ works closely with the lungs to gain oxygen and digestion to obtain nutrients.

☐ rests for a fraction of a second between beats. In a lifetime of 70 yrs. the heart rests about 40 yrs.

☐ may be harmed by emotional stress.

☐ is most active in summer.

- ☐ pumps 3000 gallons of blood a day.
- ☐ is connected to the brain and muscles. If the brain and muscles are not getting enough oxygen they send messages via the nervous system to the heart.

Humans are naturally warm blooded. The hypothalamus monitors the temperature of the blood.

Blood Pressure:

- ☐ The force of the heart muscle contraction.
- ☐ The volume of blood.
- ☐ The resistance of the blood vessels.
- ☐ The highest blood pressure is **systolic**, when the heart is pumping.
- ☐ The lowest pressure is **diastolic**, when the heart is filling up.
- ☐ Average systolic pressure is 110-120.
- ☐ Average diastolic pressure is 70-80.

HEART CONDITIONS

High blood pressure:

Treatment:

- ☐ lose weight
- ☐ eat less salt
- ☐ regular exercise
- ☐ adequate rest
- ☐ stress reduction
- ☐ reduce consumption of cigarettes, alcohol and caffeine.
- ☐ use hawthorn, garlic, cayenne and/or ginger

   Hawthorn works for both high and low blood pressure. It restores elasticity to capillary and destroys plaque. It promotes collagen production that makes the veins more elastic. Garlic works well with Hawthorn because it reduces blood pressure.

Low Blood Pressure:

- ☐ Wind - poor circulation
- ☐ Fire - equals anaemia or a damaged liver function
- ☐ Water - congestion and stagnation

HEART HEALTH

☐ One indicator of the heart's health is the tongue.

> When the heart is healthy, the tongue is moist and pink.
> When there is type A behaviour the tongue is very red.
> When the heart is weak the tongue is pale. This may show possible anaemia.
> A coated tongue relates more to digestion.

☐ A healthy heart is indicated by a rosy facial complexion and body colour, especially under fingernails.

☐ Swelling in the ankles, shin bones and under the eyes is an indicator of heart weakness.

☐ Heart weakness is also indicated by lethargy, slowness and coldness of the hands and feet.

HEART HERBS

Lily of the Valley, Hawthorn, Motherwort, Borage, Dandelion leaves.

HEART DREAMBODY

Do This!

Exercise 65 • *Nourishing Your Heart (repeat)*

Place your hand over your heart. Feel the beating of your heart. Imagine your heart sending blood full of rich oxygen and nutrition. Feel it going to every cell in your body, from the tip of your big toe to the crown of your head. Imagine all your cells bathed in this life giving fluid. Open yourself to this eternal rhythm of life affirming energy. As you breathe in imagine the blood absorbing the oxygen from your lungs and as you breathe out sense it travelling to every part of your body. When you are finished take a couple more breaths and thank your heart for its faithful work. Ask it if it needs anything? More exercise, fresh air, iron, magnesium, Vitamin E or herbs like Hawthorn, Motherwort or Lily of the Valley?

• Record your heart experience:

Do This!

Exercise 66 • *Heart Connections, The Web of Life*

Place your hand on your heart. Feel it beating while you take a couple of breaths and relax. Imagine that your heart reaches out into the world. Think about the people that you love. Imagine an invisible cord stretching from your heart to theirs. As you breath out, imagine energy travelling along this cord to them. As you breath in, imagine energy travelling back along this cord to your heart. Start with one or two people and slowly add others. As new people come to mind let the others go knowing that you are already connected. Add animals, plants, places and anything else that you feel connected to and love. When complete take a couple more breaths and thank life for all the love that you have to give and receive.

• Record your heart experience:

Small Intestine: Yang

☐ receives, digests and assimilates nourishment.
☐ sorts out and extracts the good from what we eat.
☐ is the seat of Bio-fire. In Ayurveda the word "**grahani**" refers to the active principle of the small intestine. Grahani means "that which grasps things."
    It (grahani) grasps the essence of nourishment from the food.
    It kills bacteria or pathogens in the food.

Ayurveda states that all small intestine diseases: allergies, candida, food intolerance, are best treated by healing and nourishing the small intestine.

One treatment for the small intestine is a clay poultice. If bacteria or pathogens are not killed, toxins enter the body. They cause lowered resistance, poor immune function, chronic indigestion and poor elimination. Resulting in constipation, diarrhea, gas, lack of appetite or excessive appetite, fatigue, low resistance and malabsorption syndrome. This is more common in Wind and is caused by irregular habits. In Chinese medicine it is caused by a Chi deficiency or Chi stagnation.

Blood goes straight from the small intestine to the liver. The organs support each other. Spring liver cleanse supports the small intestine in the summer.

CONSTITUTION DIFFERENTIATION FOR MAL ABSORPTION SYNDROME

Wind

Symptoms:

- [ ] Gas distention.
- [ ] Migrating pain.
- [ ] Dry skin, cracked tongue and anal fissures.
- [ ] Haemorrhoids.
- [ ] Chronic low weight.
- [ ] Tendency toward arthritis.
- [ ] Alternating constipation with diarrhoea.
- [ ] Palpitations, anxiety and insomnia.
- [ ] Feeling ungrounded and depression.

Treatment:

The anti-Wind diet. Avoid too much cold or raw food and raw juices. Consume home-made buttermilk (yoghurt and water 50/50) with fresh ginger and liquid aloe vera.

Fire

Symptoms:

- [ ] Inflammation, ulceration or burning pain in the intestines.
- [ ] Diarrhoea.
- [ ] Anaemia.
- [ ] Anger and irritability.

Treatment:

The anti-Fire diet. Avoid greasy and fried food. Take buttermilk with fennel, coriander or a bitter herb like Aloe vera.

Water

Symptoms:

- [ ] Mucus in stools.
- [ ] Dull aching pain in the abdomen.
- [ ] Heaviness.
- [ ] Congestion in the lungs.
- [ ] Edema and diabetes.

Treament: The anti-water diet. Avoid cold water, ice cream, cheese, and pastries. Take aloe juice with dry ginger or elecampane.

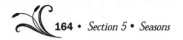

SMALL INTESTINE TONICS:

Ashwaganda, Ginseng (American or Siberian) Astragulus, Elecampane and Aloe vera.

SMALL INTESTINE DREAMBODY

Do This!

Exercise 67 • *Digesting Difficult Experiences*

Break down gross experiences into digestible ones. Remember a difficult experience that still bothers you. Write out your memory of the experience. Discuss it with a friend, in person or through the mail.

I release, lose and let go of you. "I let go and let God\Goddess" is a helpful affirmation. The Bach Flower Remedy "Willow" is a powerful ally for this process.

SUMMER ELEMENTS

Fire:

- ☐ gives light and warmth.
- ☐ maintains heat for the body
- ☐ gives warmth to others
- ☐ gives enthusiasm, vitality and energy.
- ☐ people are attracted or repulsed by the colour red.
- ☐ people thrive on activity, new ideas, ventures, adventures and change
- ☐ is YANG dominant.

  Noon is the most Yang period.

  Look out for **Yang monsters**. Yang monsters live in the fire and are very manipulative and aggressive. They will have you chasing heart attacks down the pavement in the noon day sun.

- ☐ is regulated by the bitter taste. Dandelion is a good summer bitter.

The two emotions embodied by fire and summer are joy and sadness.

☐ Joy: is light - yang.

      is manifest in the "laughing sound"

☐ Sadness: is sorrow - yin.

      is manifest in the "moaning sound"

FIRE\WATER BALANCE

Fire:	Water:
Yang	Yin
Sex\action	Feeling\receptivity
Red	Blue
Heart	Kidney

☐ **Intuition** is an attribute of the fire element.

☐ Water balances fire, internal and external. When taking water internally use filtered water.

SUMMER EXERCISE:

Do This!

Exercise 68 • *Play according to your constitution.*

Fire can be painful and intense. One of the ways of dealing with the intensity of fire in the summer is to play.

Wind: *Find an activity that gives you air and variety. Try roller skating. Be creative.*

Fire: *Go swimming or take up scuba diving. Walk by the water. Win\win games.*

Water: *Go dancing or hiking. Make exercising fun!*

FIRE:

Do This!

Exercise 69 *Fire review*

Review Fire in Ayurveda section (page 22 to 27).

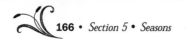

SUMMER PLANT WALK

> ### Do This!
> ### Exercise 70 • *Exploring Plants in the Summer*
> Go for a walk and observe the plants in the heat of the summer.
> Notice how different plants are responding to the fire.

SUMMER DIET

Summer is the time of year for large rainbow salads. Each colour
represents different vitamins, minerals and nutrients. Some we don't even
know about yet. By including as many different colours as we can in our diet
we assure a variety of nutrients. Sometimes the body needs one single micro-
nutrient to facilitate complex biochemical processes. Once supplied the body
gets on about it's business.

It is healthy to eat a cooling diet. My favourite food for this is celery.
The late great Dr. Christopher taught me about celery. During the hot
summers in Utah where he lived he would drink lots of celery juice. Celery
supplies organic biochemical sodium chloride that regulates the water in our
cells maintaining the proper temperature. It is helpful to cut back on heat
producing foods like proteins, dairy and starches. Favour fresh fruits and
vegetables at this time.

The most cooling taste and my favourite bitter food is Belgium endive. It
makes a great snack by itself or add to salads. A great herb to munch on, add to
salads or sandwiches is dandelion leaves. Enjoy a light diet and get outside to
play or go for long walks at this ideal time of the year.

SUMMER HERBS

Summer is usually a more playful time where I focus more on having
fun than worrying about my health. Herbs that I use are Plantain (bee stings)
Aloe Vera Gel (sunburn and sunscreen). I use Bitter, Astringent and Sweet
herbs to cool down.

Late Summer

Late summer or Indian summer is a time of seasonal transition. During this gentle abundant season, we shift our attention from the fiery expansiveness of summer toward the watery inwardness of winter. We may want to move from a lighter to a heavier diet in response to the changes of temperature.

During this time of metamorphoses it is important to stay grounded (earth element). We help achieve this through a grounded diet, staying close to the earth and using our five senses.

Do This!

Exercise 71 • *Exploring Indian Summer*

Plan to spend part of your day on or close to September 1st outside. Walk around and observe your environment. Check out the plants, animals, birds and people. Sense the play of the elements at this time.

• How do you experience the decrease of fire in your environment and body?

• How is the shortening of the day affecting your mood and sleep patterns?

LATE SUMMER BODY SYSTEMS

The two body systems associated with the late summer are the **stomach** and the **spleen**.

Stomach:

The stomach is the organ that **takes in nourishment** and begins the digestive process. It is connected to **the nervous system**, which regulates the secretion of acids and enzymes. A state of over excitement or eating too rapidly may result in digestive upset. Our eating habits connect to our energy state. Relax as you eat and savour your food. After eating relax for awhile. A short walk can aid digestion.

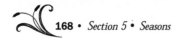

Spleen:

The spleen is the organ that distributes the energy from food. According to Chinese medicine **it rules the memory, will power and the ability to form opinions.** An imbalance in the spleen may be a lack of willpower. The spleen **governs the menstrual cycle** in women. Problems with the menstrual cycle and infertility may be caused by a spleen imbalance. The spleen **stores blood,** and **destroys old blood cells.** It is a reserve organ for blood formation.

LATE SUMMER ELEMENTS

Earth is the element of late summer. This element governs the actions of the stomach, the spleen and pancreas. The Earth element gives us the **power of manifestation.** This element connects to **forming opinions** and **creating thoughts.** An **imbalance** in the earth element may be revealed as **obsessive thinking.** Since the nervous system rules the digestive system nervous thinking may result in indigestion. Also **a strong attraction or repulsion to the colour yellow** may suggest an earth imbalance. The earth element connects to **nourishment.**

DREAMBODY HARVEST

Do This!

Exercise 72 · *Harvesting Experiences*

Take some time to think about your personal harvest. Think about any projects you have recently completed or are close to completing. Focus your attention on them and allow the experience into your body.

Allow the positive energy to renew your spirit and let go of the negative.

• Record harvest experience:

LATE SUMMER EXERCISE

Centering and becoming grounded can be part of the internal change during this transition period.

Do This!

Exercise 73 • *Using the Six Directions to Get Focussed*

Stand on the earth. Turn to the four directions and invoke their powers. Name each of the directions, North, South, East, and West. Give each direction all the attributes you think of: colour, emotion, mental characteristics and animal powers e.g. I would turn to the North and say, " I welcome in the powers of the North, coldness, clarity, wildness, wilderness, the Polar Bear, the Snow Goose and my Nordic ancestors."

Name and imagine the above, all that is above you. Next name the below, all that is below. Picture yourself surrounded by a sphere of light and energy formed by all the points of the directions. Sense and affirm yourself as the centre of this sphere. Repeat this exercise during transitions when you feel nervous or ungrounded.

• Record grounding experience:

LATE SUMMER DIET

The diet for late summer is **building and toning**. We need more fat and proteins than with the summer diet. Vegetarians would benefit from eating more whole grains and steamed vegetables. The great variety of fruits and vegetables are now coming available in the mellow days of late summer. Remember to include beans and some *dairy products. There are many ways for vegetarians to increase their protein intake such as soy, nuts and seeds. Essential minerals may be obtained from sea vegetables such as Nori, Kombu, Wakame, Hijiki, Dulse, Bladderack, Sea lettuce and many others. Meat eaters can increase their portion of poultry and fish during this time. Only increase red meat consumption a small amount.

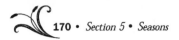

We came upon an article on milk by Robert M. Kradjian. It reduced our families consumption of dairy products to goat's milk, a little cheese and Ghee (clarified butter) To receive a copy send $3.00 to:

> Canada Earth Save Society
> #103 - 1093 W. Broadway
> Vancouver, B.C., Canada, V6H 1E2

and ask for Dr. Kradjian's Milk Letter October 1993. If you are a heavy dairy consumer I encourage you to send for it.

Fall

Fall is the season of the harvest. We gather our strength together before winter. It is a time of rich abundance, full of ripe fruits and vegetables. During the Fall we prepare for the long cold dark months of winter. The time has come for turning inward. The nights become longer than the days and we naturally begin to spend more time indoors. Fall is a good time to clear up unfinished business as we prepare internally for the change ahead of us.

Do This!
Exercise 74 • *Exploring the First Day of Fall*

Plan to spend part of your day on or close to September 21st outside. Walk around and observe your environment. Check out the plants, animals, birds and people. Sense the play of the elements at this time.

- How do you experience the decrease of fire in your environment and body?

- How is the shortening of the day affecting your mood and sleep patterns?

- Do you feel more or less energetic?

- What kind of thoughts or fantasies fill your mind during these early days of fall?

- Record Fall experiences:

FALL BODY SYSTEMS

Lungs:

The lungs connect the outer air with the inner world of the body. The lungs exchange carbon dioxide and oxygen through the pulmonary capillaries, where air and blood meet. There is external respiration through the lungs and internal respiration through the cells. The average person breathes twelve to fifteen times a minute.

Large Intestine:

The large intestine deals primarily with the elimination of solid wastes from the body. It is about five feet in length and travels around the edge of the abdomen. It is divided into the cecum, the ascending, transverse, descending and sigmoid colon. It absorbs nutrients and contains bacteria that help break down food. It forms, stores and eliminates the faeces. Food takes 24 to 36 hours to pass from mouth to anus.

The flexing of the colon is natural in childhood but becomes tempered by the early controls of school, stress, diets high in refined foods, meat and dairy. When the large intestine is congested, the organ loses its tone causing prolapses. Congestion leads to abdominal discomfort, low and mid backaches. Many backaches are connected to the large intestine.

The liver and gall bladder are important to the functioning of the intestines. When we overindulge in fried foods and alcohol our liver suffers and becomes sluggish. This impaired liver functioning slows intestinal functioning. We experience abdominal cramps in the morning, a stiff back and sinus congestion. A diet of natural foods, grains and steamed vegetables will keep the intestines working well. Regular exercise like walking is important.

Immune System:

Defines me from not me. It destroys harmful "not me's" such as harmful bacteria and viruses. Ayurveda personifies it, calling it Ahamkara, our joy and will to live.

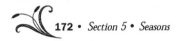

DREAMBODY IMMUNE SYSTEM

I include this in Wind season as we are most easily influenced at this time. It is time to prepare ourselves for the challenges of winter. When you move away from the direction of your dreams we find that people tend to get sick easier. Remember you only need to move 1/4 inch in the direction of your dreams to start feeling better. Bernard Jensen use to say, "You have got to feel good, to feel good."

Do This!

Exercise 75 • *Stimulating the Immune System with Lighter Dreams*

If your life is not up to what you had hoped it would be, then imagine a more optimistic and desirable future for your self! Play with this vision. Meditate on it. Write it down. Draw it. Allow it to permeate your cells. Imagine how you would move if your life was like this dream. Think about some small steps that you might take towards manifesting this life.

• Record your experience:

BALANCING THE CONSTITUTIONS

Pacify the constitution disturbed (likely Wind). Wind brings Fire and Water into line. Treat Wind with rest, meditation, warmth and massage.

We treat congestion first if present.

WIND (VATA)

Do This!

Exercise 76 • *Review Wind (Vata)*

Review the section on Wind in the Ayurveda section. (page 22 to 27)

FALL ELEMENTS

In the Chinese system of healing **Metal** is the element of Fall. This is the element of mental activity. In Ayurveda the element of Fall is Air that represents the mind and communication.

AIR SPIRIT

"Outside the air bubble (atmosphere) are the dead. Air power can't be accepted until you earn it. Pray all the time. Communicate through the air power. Daybreak is the best time. It makes your mind inquisitive. It makes the difference between living and thriving." Ellen White.

Do This!
Exercise 77 • *Corralling Air Power*

Go outside when you wake up. Greet the world and ask for forgiveness. Ask the air "have we done anything to offend you?" Tell it, "We love you, help us to be strong. We thank you." (Never use I.) Talk to your body. Feel the air power going through you. Collect air power. Do this daily for a week.

It is helpful but not necessary to drink cleansing teas like Red Clover, Dandelion and\or Yellow Dock, 3 or 4 days a week to make you more receptive.

• Record your experience:

FALL ENERGY

September 21st (approx.) marks Fall Equinox. At this time the light and the dark are equal. From now on the dark time will be increasing and the light decreasing. Many indigenous cultures celebrate the equinoxes and solstices, acknowledging the shift in energy as we go through waxing, peaking and waning of the light. I marvel at the magic of this planet spinning perfectly through space and gently shifting on its axis, creating the seasons.

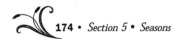

In Fall the Yin cycle begins. Yin energy is similar to Water. In the northern climates it is cold, wet, dark, heavy (falls to the earth) and inward (keeps many of us inside or makes us more introspective). Beware of Yin monsters. Yin monsters live in the water and are very seductive. They may have you passively crying in your soup before you realize it. We need to strengthen our Yin and sometimes that means slowing down, turning inward and dealing with some of our internal demons. **Following this natural ebb and flow of the seasons makes our life easier and more rewarding.**

FALL PLANT WALK

Do This!
Exercise 78 • *Observing the Plants in the Fall*
Go out and observe the local plants in the Fall. Notice how they respond to the energy of Fall.

FALL HERBS

In the fall we need herbs that reduce excess wind. These are the carminatives, nervines, demulcents and laxatives. The oil from **Borage, Flax and Evening Primrose** are excellent at this time. **Ginger** can be added to soups and teas. **Valerian** is an excellent earthy nervine for any wind types that need help feeling grounded and need help sleeping. **Marshmallow** is very nourishing, moistening and soothing to the body. **Castor oil** is good for troubles with constipation.

FALL DIET

The diet for Fall is **building and toning.** We need more fat and proteins now. Vegetarians would benefit from eating more whole grains and steamed vegetables. Remember to include beans and dairy products (highest quality you can find). There are many other ways for vegetarians to increase their protein intake such as legumes, soy, nuts and seeds. Essential minerals may be obtained from sea vegetables such as Nori, Kombu, Wakame, Hijiki, Dulse, Bladderack, Sea lettuce and many others. B12 supplementation may benefit strict vegetarians.

Winter

This is the season when water is the dominant element. It is the time of feelings, a deep **Yin time**. Winter is the time to replenish yourself and bring all the constitutions into balance. This is the best time to rest and search for the clarity you need to visualize the year ahead. Use the flow chart and the flow paradigm to help you in making your choices.

Do This!

Exercise 79 • *Exploring the First Day of Winter*

Plan to spend part of your day on or close to December 21st outside. Walk around and observe your environment. Check out the plants, animals, birds and people. Sense the play of the elements at this time.

- How do you experience the decrease of fire in your environment and body?

- How is the shortening of the day affecting your mood and sleep patterns?

- Do you feel more or less energetic?

- What kind of thoughts or fantasies fill your mind during these early days of winter?

WINTER ACTIVITIES

Dreaming

Dream time is very important. Winter was the season indigenous cultures went inside to dream, dance and enact their rituals. In the Pacific Northwest where I live, the natives have their bighouse for this purpose. Winter is naturally a time we have less light and warmth to tempt us outside. It is healthy to go with the natural rhythm of the season. Find a cosy spot to **relax, sleep and dream.**

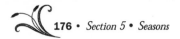

Go to bed early and get up late. Seek inner warmth with family and friends. Keep warm (especially the kidneys). Communicate your feelings. Ayurveda suggests that it is the best time for sexual relations. A healing activity for body and soul.

Childhood Dream

> ### *Do This!*
> ### Exercise 80 • *Redo Childhood Dream*
> Winter would be a good time to redo the childhood dream exercise from the introduction. (see page 10)

WINTER BODY SYSTEMS

Kidneys:	Bladder:
YIN	YANG
seat of the will	storehouse of the emotions
lack of will or ambition	stretching the back opens meridians
may represent water imbalance	
Where the Chi (vital energy) is stored	
5-7 pm. filling time	3-5 pm. filling time

The bladder meridian (adrenals) turns off and on again at will. It sends energy to the brain and regulates body energy. In Chinese medicine a deficiency in the water element equals an inability to slow down and an inability to think clearly. When the water element is in balance there is fluidity and flow. There is an ability to rest and nourish the self and others. The water element guides perception and reflection. With the water element in balance there is a ready expression of feelings like love and compassion. Attraction or repulsion to the colour blue may show a water imbalance.

Urine: a waste product of the body can be a good indicator of health.

Blackish brown = Wind disorder	Dark yellow = Fire disorder
Cloudy = Water disorder	Foul smell = toxins
Sweet = excess sugar	Gravel = possible stones
Green = excess bile	Clear urine = too much water.

Kidneys:

>Excrete and conserve water.
>
>Eliminate toxins.
>
>Return water, salt, potassium and other vital substances to the blood in just the right amount to keep the body's internal environment stable.
>
>Time: Filling at 5:00 PM. to 7:00 PM.
>
>Taste: Salty
>
>Emotion: Fear and Anxiety.

GINGER COMPRESS

Kidney tonic and cleanse

Dissolve one half a cup of powdered ginger in two quarts of hot water. Soak a small towel in the solution and place it on the kidney area, just at the base of the ribs. Take care not to burn the patient! Cover the damp towel up with other towels or a blanket. Keep the back warm while massaging the hands or feet to open the meridians.

This compress feels wonderfully relaxing and nurturing to the kidneys. Take care not to send the patient out into the cold immediately afterward. Be sure they are dressed warm.

Warning: This treatment moves toxins caused by congestion through the body. Some people experience various symptoms afterward. These symptoms pass quickly.

Warning!   **Do not apply compress if there is pain, infection or damage to the kidneys.**

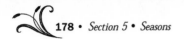

DREAMBODY KIDNEYS

> ### *Do This!*
> ### Exercise 81 • *Exploring the Body Dreams in our Kidneys*
> Lay down somewhere comfortable on your stomach. Ask a
> friend to place their hand on your kidneys (at the base of your
> ribs). Focus your attention where their hand is. Take a few
> minutes to absorb your attention into this area. Now dream
> about your ancestors and let your mind drift back into your
> family's past. Go back to the land or lands that your family
> came from.
>
> Ask your ancestors for guidance and help with your life
> mission. Feel all the power of your ancestors concentrated in
> this area of your body. When you feel the energy has built up
> enough, then spread it to the rest of your body. Feel it move
> from your kidneys and spread to all parts of your body from
> your head to your toes. Thank your ancestors. Now share your
> experience with your assistant.

The Chinese consider the kidneys as home of our ancestral chi (energy,
life force).

WATER (Kapha)

> ### *Do This!*
> ### Exercise 82 • *Review Water*
> Winter is a good time to review Water in the Ayurveda section.
> (see page 22 to 28)

Do This!

Exercise 83 • *Journeying with a Drum*

Find a comfortable place where you won't be disturbed. Either have an assistant drum for you or use a drum tape. The drum should be at 180 beats per minute. A little faster or slower beat may be necessary for you to journey. We often use a deer skin drum. Shamans traditionally use the deer spirit to enter the spirit world. Deer spirit allows us to leave and arrive safely.

Take a few breaths to get comfortable. Remember an opening in the earth, a vortex, pool or pond. This will be your entry point. When going on a journey, remember that whatever happens during the journey is right. Descend into the opening and follow whatever opens up before you. If you are offered anything to bring back, we encourage you to decline. If you can't enter the opening right away, relax and enjoy the drum and begin when ready. If you meet a block or obstruction simply come back and try again. It becomes easier with practice.

Most journeys last under fifteen minutes. The tape or assistant will call you back with four short strong beats, followed by a sucession of rapid beats. Keep a record of your journeys in a journal.

THE YIN\YANG-LIGHT\DARK CYCLE

Winter is the darkest time of the year. Many of us need extra natural light to keep our pituitary gland functioning at normal levels. It is a time when some people suffer S.A.D.'s (Seasonal Affective Disorder). They suffer depression that is only corrected by increasing the amount of light that they receive each day. They get up a couple of hours early and sit under some form of full spectrum lighting. I also encourage people to get outside in the natural light as much as they can.

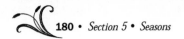

WINTER EMOTIONS

Feelings are dominant in winter.

> ### *Do This!*
> **Exercise 84** • *Winter Feelings*
> Redo the feeling path exercises from page 120. This is the best season to get in touch with your feelings.

WINTER EXERCISE

Water needs to stay in motion. Some good winter exercises are walking, dance, yoga, Feldenkrais, Tai Chi and stretching.

WINTER PLANT WALK

> ### *Do This!*
> **Exercise 85** • *Observing the Plants in Winter*
> Go out and observe the local plants in winter. Notice how they adapt to the winter conditions.

WINTER DIET

Concentrate on warming foods. Root vegetables are perfect as they reflect the energy of the season, underground and inward. Grains and beans, tofu, fish or a small amount of red meat supply protein for body warmth. Aduki beans are especially good as they are a kidney tonic. Seaweeds contain a rich source of the many minerals we need. Soups are ideal at this time of year, hot and nutritious. Milk is best warm with a little pungent herb like Cinnamon or Ginger. Honey is a good sweetener in the winter but it should not be heated. This is a great time to enjoy warm herbal teas. Add spices, gomasio (sesame salt) or tamari (soya sauce) to your food. Reduce or avoid table salt. Eat less fruit at this time.

Do This!

Exercise 86 • *Muscle Response Test*

Muscle test to see what the body prefers. Muscle testing involves putting the thumb and pinky finger together. The next step is to ask the body about a type of food while attempting to pull the two digits apart. If the food or substance is needed by the body then there will be strong resistance. If the food is not useful or harmful the digits will come apart easily.

WINTER HERBS

Depending on what your winters are like, we tend to favour Pungent, Bitter and Astringent Herbs during our cold damp winters. My favourites are Ginger, Garlic, Elecampane, Echinacea, Propolis, Coffee and Yarrow.

Your Notes:

Section 6
Conclusion

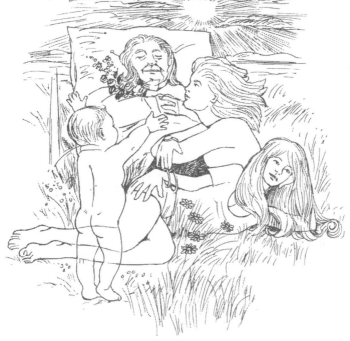

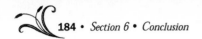

Flow, Purpose and Order

*Ayurveda, Flow and the Seasons
give us a very strong framework to work and live within,
helping us to maintain order and wellness.*

This section deals with some of the larger issues of our life, like our life's purpose. How to set up a lifestyle that facilitates flow instead of congestion. How we sometimes need to go through chaos to find a new order. In the lesson I have listed four books for your further study.

After this section you will be able to:
1) define the eight elements of flow and apply them to some of your own life projects.
2) explain why crisis may be necessary for change.
3) begin exploring your life purpose.

THE FLOW PARADIGM

The Flow Paradigm, helps us define **which activities affirm life** and **which are depleting.** If any activity does not flow, chances are, your life force will be depleted by it. In our goal of well being, it is important for us to be aware of the effect that the life we are creating has on our well being. **I use this system regularly** to monitor my activities to the betterment of my short and long term wellness.

The following is a condensation of the basic elements of the flow paradigm as laid out in the book "Flow, The Psychology of Optimal Experience" by Mihaly Csikszentmihalyi.

THE EIGHT ELEMENTS OF FLOW:

☐ Challenge:
Is the challenge difficult enough to make us grow but reasonable enough to complete?
Do we possess the right skills and proper tools to complete it?
The levels of Challenge

• Boring	•• Duty
••• Exciting	•••• Very exciting

One can alter challenges by: changing ones attitude, adding or deleting certain aspects. This may be necessary when one temporarily sticks to a boring situation.

☐ **Time and space:**

Do we have the time and freedom to concentrate on the task?

☐ **Clear goals:**

Is the goal clear? " No favourable winds blow for a ship that has no port."

☐ **Feedback:**

Is there fairly immediate and desirable feedback (a compliment, some encouragement, a good feeling, excitement)?

☐ **Depth:**

Is this activity compelling enough to remove us from the worries and frustrations of everyday life?

☐ **Control:**

Does this activity give you a sense of control over your actions?

☐ **Self:**

Does your sense of self get lost while engaged in the activity and emerges stronger after the experience?

☐ **Time Sense:**

Does the activity alter your sense of time?

Do This!

Exercise 87 • *Exploring the Flow Paradigm*

Run a few of your personal projects through this paradigm to see how they flow according to this model. Are they challenging enough? Do you have enough time and space to work on them? Is your goal clear? What kind of feedback are you receiving? Is it stimulating enough to keep you going? When working on it do you feel removed from your everyday world? Are you growing from it?

LIFE PURPOSE

According to Larry Dossey the number one illness that takes more lives than all other disease is heart disease. The number one cause of heart disease is job dissatisfaction. Most strokes occur at 9:00 am. on Monday morning. We are the only species that has managed to cluster a specific disease at a specific time.

Dr. Bach was right-on when he narrowed down the major causes of disease to two areas. The first was not following your path (life purpose - Wild oat). The second was harming others (love - Holly).

Since this area cuts to the heart of health and well being I recommend the two following books. The first is "**How to Find your Mission in Life**" by R.N. Bolles. In it he emphasises your **uniqueness** as crucial if you are ever to find meaningful work. Finding your life mission is a search of the **heart as** well as the mind. It is a **deep mystery** that needs time to unfold. The search is a **learning process. It will involve making the world a better place.** In Ellen White's mythology, the Creator did the best job He could but He needs **our constant feedback to improve creation.** We need to find our unique mission that uses our **particular gifts**, that we **delight in using**, in the **place(s) or setting(s) that appeal to us most**. I find the clue of place and setting helpful.

You may get involved in a career like herbalism because you love to be in nature and then find yourself working downtown in a store. I have loved nature all my life and I like to spend as much time outside as I can. In fact, I need to, to maintain normal functioning of my pituitary gland. After considering the above we then need to look for **the work that most needs doing.**

It is an unlearning process as well as a learning process. We need to unlearn the idea that our purpose is to keep busy doing something. Re-learn to spend time **BEING** something. **Vervain** Bach flower remedy is good for this state. Let go of the notion that everything about our work must be unique to us. Learn that some portion of our mission we share with all life. We need to change our notion that our unique mission must consist of some achievement that all the world will see. That what we have accomplished is our doing, and ours alone. We all stand on the backs of each other.

At some point you may experience some grand mountain top experience. You say to yourself "This, this, is why I came into the world. I know it." Until then, your mission is here in the valley and the fog. The little callings, that happen moment to moment and day to day. The work that fulfills us, is **where our deep-seated joy and the world's buried hunger meet.**

The second book I found helpful in this area is, *Do What you Love and the Money will Follow* by M. Sinetar. Be sure to read her second book *To Build the Life You Want, Create the Work You Love* before making any major changes. She believes that people can fulfill themselves as authentic, unique human beings through doing their right livelihoods. As people respect the venture they value most, by doing it, they become more authentic, reliable and self-disciplined. They grow to trust themselves more. It is inner listening that is necessary if one wants to follow "**the way of the heart**" to the work that is most enjoyable and fulfilling. Doing what one loves provides rich **inner rewards** that include money but also transcend money.

Work needs to fit your personality just as shoes fit your feet. Otherwise you are destined for discomfort. **Right work is just as important to personal health and growth as the right nutrients are for our bodies.** People who are successful **enjoy their work.** They enjoy it in part **because they are good at it.** Any talent that we are born with eventually surfaces as a need. Turning our lives around is usually the beginning of maturity since it means correcting choices made unconsciously, without deliberation or thought. Once we see and accept that **our talents are also our blueprint for a satisfying vocational life**, then we can stop looking to others for approval and direction.

Our enjoyment predisposes us to create more and better works and enables others to see value in them. They value us with the trust, respect and money that support our efforts. Almost anyone who devotes herself to a given vocation by pouring her love and energy into that activity, develops a certain **genius** in that field. The vocation opens itself up to her in terms of its truths and principles. It bends itself to her imagery and ideas. It **becomes her friend** and most able co-creator. As she invests herself in the work she grows. She works because she is in love with what she does.

She senses in an intuitive, strange way that **the work loves her too** and opens itself up to her. It shows her its special rules, secrets and requirements. She grows to see that her work is more than something by which to "earn a living." It is **that which helps her build a life.**

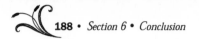

Do This!

Exercise 88 • *Exploring Your Life Purpose*

Reflect on and answer the following questions. Be gentle with yourself as this is a large undertaking. One study showed improved immune response by those attempting to find their life purpose even if they failed to achieve it. Trying was healthier than not trying. Some statistics report that 95% of the North American population do not enjoy what they are doing. I think that is way too high!

• What is unique about yourself and your skills?

• What do you enjoy doing?

• What is your favourite place or setting?

• What do you see as something that needs to be done that someone else is not doing or they are not able to do it all or do it well enough?

• Who do you envy and what are they doing that you might want to be doing?

• Have you had any strong dreams that may point to a certain direction?

When you get some ideas of the sort of work you would like to do, then invite it into your heart and see how it feels. Begin taking small steps toward it, e.g. Go to the library and take out some books on the subject.

• Record your life purpose experience:

Attention

Applied awareness is the outward expression of our soul.

Attention is our **primary tool for healing, growth and transformation.** The information we allow into consciousness determines the content and quality of life. Information enters consciousness because we focus on it or because of attentional habits. Our attention selects appropriate pieces of information from the millions of pieces available. We retrieve the appropriate references from memory, to evaluate an event and then choose the right course of action.

Some of us learn to use attention efficiently; others waste it. The mark of a person proficient with consciousness is the ability to focus attention at will. To be oblivious to distractions and concentrate as long as it takes to achieve a goal and not longer. You can develop this skill through the exercises in the Pathways to Healing.

Whenever information disrupts consciousness by threatening its goals we have a condition of inner disorder, or psychic entropy. Prolonged experiences of this kind can weaken us to the point where we can no longer invest attention and pursue our goals. We move away from the edges of our personal growth. We will learn how to pick up our edges, process new information and stay on our path.

ORDER OUT OF CHAOS
Dissipated Structure

The term dissipated structure was coined by a Belgian chemist Ilya Prigogine to describe fluctuations in a system that causes new complexity. This idea was brought to bear on human health in "Time Space and Medicine" by Dr. Larry Dossey.

Life manifests a "shake-up" or some kind of crisis to our original structure, such as sickness to our normally healthy body. The disruption is a **reordering opportunity.** It occurs in any system, such as a company, institution, country, relationship, or our bodies. The Chinese character for **"crises"** means both danger and opportunity.

The thought of a crisis fills most of us with fear. Yet the institution or person that never changes may begin to stagnate. A **key to growth** is to flow and work with disturbances. Good art disturbs us into a new way of thinking. In Nature our bodies' fine-tuned sophisticated immune systems are exposed to disease and disruption. We need to find ways to let go of old patterns and structures, when faced with crises, so we can grow and achieve new order. The new order is stronger and more adaptable. This idea is a new and healthy way of looking at our life's shake-ups, accidents and diseases.

DON'S PARADIGM OF HEALING

Treat the person not the disease! When consulting listen to the first couple of things that they say to you and write them down. Be sure that you address these points. Figure out what constitution they are and which constitution is disturbed? Consider whether the constitution in question is with or without congestion.

Feedback:

It is vital to watch and or feel for feedback . This may be difficult because of the many factors affecting you. It is beneficial to start with few interventions at first so you can figure out which ones are working. Remember that some of the more nutritive herbs need some time to manifest their benefit. The goal is to strengthen the person and reduce their symptoms. If working with someone else, involve the patient by **educating** her and have her modify her treatment according to **her body's feedback.**

Change:

Encourage small changes to their habits and routines that help balance out the constitution. These can become restful routines. i.e.

☐ Wind - a hot bath in the **late afternoon.**
☐ Fire - go for a swim or take a walk by some water around **noon.**
☐ Water - vigorous exercise in the **morning** (before noon).

Encourage according to the Constitution.

☐ Wind - make it **exciting**. Only one or two changes.
☐ Fire - make it **challenging** and transformational.
☐ Water - make it resourceful and **stimulating.**

Support:

☐ Ask the patient to involve a friend or loved one in their healing process.

Growth:

☐ Ask them what is right about their problem? Help them to become aware of different parts that may be resisting change. Process their symptom using technique in dreambody section. Make their symptom an Ally (helper).

Refer back to the section The Art of Practicing Herbalism on page 97 for including herbs.

Death & Rebirth

Since we have been studying cycles and seasons we cannot move forward without a word about death. In some cultures a person is not trained in healing until they are comfortable with death. One of the best books that I read on death was The Mystery of Death by Kirpal Singh. Stephen Levine and Elizabeth Kubler Ross also address the subject well in their writings.

After this lesson you will be able to:
1) write your own epitaph.
2) using a dying process to help you make changes.

LIVING AND DYING

As we dance with life, life dances with us. Sometimes the dance is smooth and flowing, sometimes jagged and tense. Sometimes it becomes stuck. Movement is life and stagnation is death, death of the cell and death of the self. Death can be an ally. Sometimes it is important for parts of us to die.

When the dance becomes stuck it may be time for a death. It may be time to go within and connect with the part of us that wants to die and help it to die. With death comes rebirth.

Some deaths are easier than others. When I think of changing my profession, edge-figures opposed to that change, activate. They have a 25-year investment in keeping me in the same profession.

Seasons have deaths. When we pass the Winter Solstice, the light will be on the increase. At that time, it is time to begin dying to the darkness and embrace the increasing light.

Fear of death is accompanied by an identity crisis. Change your identity and the fears goes. There may be a rejuvenating effect from fantasizing our deaths and getting on with our changes.

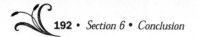

Do This!

Exercise 89 • *Composing Your own Epitaph*

Write out your epitaph. See if you are happy with it. If not, consider making the necessary changes in your life, as you have no guarantee how long you will live.

• Record your epitaphs:

Do This!

Exercise 90 • *Journey to Rebirth*

Have a close friend guide you through a death and rebirth. Lay down and imagine that you are dying. Follow the fantasy through the stages of death and whatever follows. Notice what part of you wants to die? Let yourself die, just for a minute. What part wants to be born? Embrace that part and experience what it feels like. What part may be resisting the change or death (the edge figure, the blocker)?

Pick up the role of the edge figure. Work with the edge figure by having a dialogue him\her and role playing with your assistant. Try to understand the edge figure by occupying his or her role. See if you can figure out what they want or need. Maybe make some kind of deal with them. The closer you stay to your growing edges the more alive you will feel.

• Record your dying experiences:

ALCHEMY

Alchemy
    a piece of earth
    a body of water
    a touch of fire.

Searching for the healing
    the knowledge
    the contact
    with the elemental powers.

How does the touch of fire,
    the feel of earth,
    the flow of water
    connect to the herbs?

I observe the leaves
    growing from the earth
    remember the recent rains
    fire's touch sprouts these plants.

Consider the connection of:
    the elements
    the plants
    the tastes
    our bodies
    our dreams

Smelling the earth
    I enter a joyful trance.
    the odour permeates
    my bones
    my marrow.

Water
    as I ride your waves.
    I come to know
    your Neptune ways,
    the storms
    the calm.

Fire
    as I touch and I am touched
    by your gentle and fierce heat
    I move toward the sun
    like a moth to the flame
    consumer and consumed.

Wind
    I hear you in the trees.
    watch you ripple
    through their leaves.

Planet Earth, our school, our
    playground, our home.

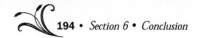

Appendix #1

CATNIP Nepeata cataria

Dosage: Strong infusion- 1/2 to 1 cup 2 to5 x day before meals
Tincture- 2 to 5 ml. 2 to 5 x day before meals

CHAMOMILE Matricaria chamomilla

Dosage: Strong infusion- 1/2 to 1 cup 2 to5 x day before meals
Tincture- 2 to 5 ml. 2 to 5 x day before meals

HOPS Humulus lupulus

Dosage: Mild infusion- 1/2 to 1 cup 2 to5 x day after meals
Tincture- 1 to 2 ml. 2 to 5 x day after meals

LEMON VERBENA Verbena

Dosage: Strong infusion- 1/2 to 1 cup 2 to 5 x day after meals
Tincture- 2 to 5 ml. 2 to 5 x day after meals

SKULLCAP Scutellaria latiflora

Dosage: Strong infusion- 1/2 to 1 cup 2 to 5 x day after meals
Tincture- 2 to 5 ml. 2 to 5 x day after meals

VALERIAN ROOT Valarian officinalis

Dosage: Strong infusion- 1/2 to 1 cup 2 to 5 x day after meals
Tincture- 2 to 5 ml. 2 to 5 x day after meals

VERVAIN Verbena officinalis

Dosage: Strong infusion- 1/2 to 1 cup 2 to 5 x day after meals
Tincture- 2 to 5 ml. 2 to 5 x day after meals

SAINT JOHNSWORT Hypericum perforatum

Dosage: Tincture- 3 to 5 ml. 3 to 5 x day
Allow at least 6 weeks for full affect

BLUE COHOSH ROOT Caulophyllum thralietroides

Dosage: Decoction- 1/2 to 1 cup 2 to 5 x day before meals
Tincture- 2 to 5 ml. 2 to 5 x day before meals

SHEPHERD'S PURSE Capsella bursa-pastoris
Dosage: Strong infusion- 1/2 to 1 cup 2 to 5 x day after meals
Tincture- 2 to 5 ml. 2 to 5 x day after meals

CRAMPBARK Viburnum opulus
Dosage: Decoction- 1/2 to 1 cup 2 to 5 x day before meals
Tincture- 2 to 5 ml. 2 to 5 x day before meals

BLACK COHOSH ROOT Cimifuga racemosa
Dosage: Decoction- 1/2 to 1 cup 2 to 5 x day before meals
Tincture- 2 to 5 ml. 2 to 5 x day before meals

CHICKWEED Stellaria media
Dosage: Strong infusion-1/2 to 1 cup 2 to 5 x day before meals
Tincture- 2 to 5 ml. 2 to 5 x day before meals

CALENDULA FLOWERS Calendula officinalis
Dosage: Strong infusion-1/2 to 1 cup 2 to 5 x day before meals
Tincture- 2 to 5 ml. 2 to 5 x day before meals

WALNUT HULLS Juglans nigra
Dosage: Strong infusion-1/2 to 1 cup 2 to 5 x day before meals
Tincture- 2 to 5 ml. 2 to 5 x day before meals

GOLDENSEAL ROOT Hydrastis canadensis
Dosage: Strong infusion-1/2 to 1 cup 2 to 5 x day before meals
Tincture- 2 to 5 ml. 2 to 5 x day before meals

MARSHMALLOW ROOT Althea officinalis
Dosage: Strong infusion-1/2 to 1 cup 2 to 5 x day before meals
Tincture- 2 to 5 ml. 2 to 5 x day before meals

MYRRH Commiphora myrrha
Dosage: Tincture- 5 to 15 drops 2 to 5 x day before meals

MULLEIN FLOWERS Verbascum thapsus
Dosage: Strong infusion-1/2 to 1 cup 2 to 5 x day after meals
Tincture- 2 to 5 ml. 2 to 5 x day after meals

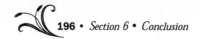

ECHINACEA Echinacea angustifolia or purpurea

Dosage: Decoction-1/2 to 1 cup 2 to 5 x day before meals
Tincture- 2 to 5 ml. 2 to 5 x day before meals

PROPOLIS

Dosage: Tincture- 5 to 15 drops in a glass of warm water (some resin may stick to glass, alcohol can be used to clean it) gargle if your throat is sore and then swallow
Capsules: for stomach ulcers I fill "00" capsules with 15 drops of tincture and use immediately. 1 or 2 capsules before meals.

GARLIC Allium sativum

Dosage: Tincture- 2 to 5 ml. 2 to 5 x day before meals
Capsules- 1 cap 2 to 5 x day before meals

DEVIL'S CLAW ROOT Harpagophytum procumbens

Dosage: Decoction- 1/2 to 1 cup 2 to 5 x day before meals
Tincture- 2 to 5 ml. 2 to 5 x day before meals

FEVERFEW Tanacetum parthenium

Dosage: Mild infusion- 1/2 to 1 cup 2 to 5 x day before meals
Tincture- 1 to 2 ml. 2 to 5 x day before meals
Chewing a couple of fresh leaves a day works
To abort a migrain take every 15 minutes up to 3 times

GENTIAN ROOT Gentiana lutea

Dosage: Mild infusion- 1/2 to 1 cup 2 to 5 x day before meals
Tincture- 1 to 2 ml. 2 to 5 x day before meals

YARROW Achillea millefolium

Dosage: Strong infusion- 1/2 to 1 cup 2 to 5 x day before meals
Tincture- 2 to 5 ml. 2 to 5 x day before meals

PEPPERMINT Mentha piperita

Dosage: Strong infusion- 1/2 to 1 cup 2 to 5 x day before meals
Tincture- 2 to 5 ml. 2 to 5 x day before meals

GINGER ROOT Zingiber officinale

Dosage: Strong infusion- 1/2 to 1 cup 2 to 5 x day before meals
Tincture (weak)- 1 to 2 ml. 2 to 5 x day before meals

DAMIANA Turnera aphrodissiaca

Dosage: Strong infusion- 1/2 to 1 cup 2 to 5 x day before meals
Tincture- 2 to 5 ml. 2 to 5 x day before meals

MUGWORT Artimisia vulgaris

Dosage: Strong infusion- 1/2 to 1 cup 2 to 5 x day before meals
Tincture- 1 to 3 ml. 2 to 5 x day before meals

PENNYROYAL Mentha pulegium

Dosage: Strong infusion- 1/2 to 1 cup 2 to 5 x day before meals
Tincture- 1 to 3 ml. 2 to 5 x day before meals

BUCHU Agathosma betulina

Dosage: Strong infusion- 1/2 to 1 cup 2 to 5 x day before meals
Tincture- 2 to 4 ml. 2 to 5 x day before meals

CLEAVERS Gallium aparine

Dosage: Strong infusion- 1/2 to 1 cup 2 to 5 x day before meals
Tincture- 2 to 5 ml. 2 to 5 x day before meals

JUNIPER BERRIES Juniperus communis

Dosage: Strong infusion- 1/2 to 1 cup 2 to 5 x day before meals
Tincture- 1 to 2 ml. 2 to 5 x day before meals

PIPSISSEWA Chimaphila umbellata

Dosage: Strong infusion- 1/2 to 1 cup 2 to 5 x day before meals
Tincture- 2 to 5 ml. 2 to 5 x day before meals

ELECAMPANE ROOT Inula helenium

Dosage: Decoction- 1/2 to 1 cup 2 to 5 x day after meals
Tincture- 2 to 5 ml. 2 to 5 x day after meals

DEVIL'S CLUB BARK OF ROOT Oplopanax horridus

Dosage: Decoction- 1/2 to 1 cup 2 to 5 x day before meals
Tincture- 2 to 5 ml. 2 to 5 x day before meals

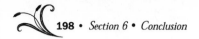

Index

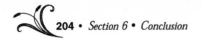

DON OLLSIN

Don Ollsin is a pioneering educator and leading practitioner in the field of herbal medicine. His story begins in 1969 when, working in Vancouver's Golden Lotus Restaurant as one of B.C.'s first vegetarian chefs, his inherent love of natural food drew him to the study of herbs and their therapeutic value. At this time he began to apprentice under the noted American herbal authority Dr. John Christopher with whom he studied the science and art of herbalism. Wanting to work directly in the natural health field, he moved to Victoria, B.C. in 1972 and opened Sawan Natural Foods, which included Victoria's first herbal dispensary.

In 1976, Don began to study through the Emerson Institute of Herbal Studies. That same year he decided to devote all his energies to promoting the value of herbal medicine and opened Self Heal Herbs in Victoria, a retail store and information resource centre which helped to set the guidelines for quality herbal medicine and education. Don received his Master Herbalist's degree from the Emerson Institute and soon after began teaching classes on herbs and healing, eventually broadening his activities to include lecturing and giving workshops with noted authors and teachers. Don has been an active member of the Canadian Herbalist Association of B.C. since 1977.

As a professional herbalist with a practical orientation, Don believes in seeing results. His knowledge of what works comes from his years of experience in treating the widest range of conditions among his thousands of clients. In 1987, Don began to offer an intensive herbal training program called the Herbal Healing Journey and also developed a home study program. In the fall of 1996 Don began teaching at the Division of Continuing Studies of the University of Victoria, where he created the course entitled "Western and Local Herbs for Healing."

Don believes that herbs have a place in today's evolving health care system. He would like to see more herbal education in the public schools, in colleges and in universities. He wants to see more people learning about herbs grown in their local area and how to work with them with care and respect. He envisions the development of community-based herbal medicine in which the majority of the medicinal herbs used are grown and produced by the communities they serve.

Don continues his work as a herbal consultant at Self Heal Herbs in Victoria. In January of 1998 he began the Practical (Earth-based) Herbalist Program at Langara College in Vancouver. He also teaches herbal classes at the University of Victoria.

Book Orders:

PATHWAYS TO HEALING

herbalhealingpathway.com

or

1-800-852-4890

Courses:

PRACTICAL HERBALIST CERTIFICATE PROGRAM

CONSULTANT HERBALIST CERTIFICATE PROGRAM

HERBAL HEALING PROGRAMS VIA THE INTERNET

herbalhealingpathway.com

healing@herbalhealingpathway.com

Book Orders:

PATHWAYS TO HEALING

herbalhealingpathway.com

or

1-800-852-4890

Courses:

PRACTICAL HERBALIST CERTIFICATE PROGRAM

CONSULTANT HERBALIST CERTIFICATE PROGRAM

HERBAL HEALING PROGRAMS VIA THE INTERNET

herbalhealingpathway.com

healing@herbalhealingpathway.com